Procedures in Phlebotomy

Edited by

John C. Flynn, Jr., Ph.D., M.S., M.T. (ASCP) S.B.B.

Director, Medical Laboratory Technician and
    Phlebotomy Programs
Montgomery County Community College
Blue Bell, Pennsylvania

W.B. SAUNDERS COMPANY
A Division of Harcourt Brace & Company
Philadelphia   London   Toronto   Montreal   Sydney   Tokyo

W. B. Saunders Company
A Division of Harcourt Brace & Company

The Curtis Center
Independence Square West
Philadelphia, Pennsylvania 19106

Library of Congress Cataloging-in-Publication Data

Procedures in phlebotomy/edited by John C. Flynn, Jr.
   p.   cm.
  ISBN 0-7216-4685-9
  1. Phlebotomy.   I. Flynn, John C.,
  [DNLM: 1. Blood Specimen Collection — methods. 2. Bloodletting —
methods.   WB 381 P963 1994]
  RM182.P76   1994
  616.07′561 — dc20
  DNLM/DLC   93-26278
  for Library of Congress

Procedures in Phlebotomy   ISBN 0-7216-4685-9

Printed in the United States of America

Last digit is the print number: 9   8   7   6   5   4   3   2

I would like to dedicate this book to my
wife, Mary Ellen, and our children,
Meghan, Mary Ellen, Jack, Eamonn, Rory,
and Brighid.

Contributors

Barbara Janson Cohen, B.A., M.S.
Instructor, Delaware County Community College,
Media, Pennsylvania; Lecturer, Thomas Jefferson
University, Philadelphia, Pennsylvania
Anatomy and Physiology

Georganne K. Buescher, M.S., Ed.D.
Instructor, Department of Microbiology and
Immunology, Jefferson Medical College, Thomas
Jefferson University, Philadelphia, Pennsylvania;
Director of Master of Science Programs, College of
Graduate Studies (Microbiology and Biomedical
Chemistry), and Associate Dean, College of Graduate
Studies, Thomas Jefferson University, Philadelphia,
Pennsylvania
Infectious Diseases and Their Prevention

Beth V. Dronson, V.M.D.
Associate Veterinarian, Warminster Veterinary
Hospital, Warminster, Pennsylvania
Animal Phlebotomy

John C. Flynn, Jr., Ph.D., M.S., M.T.(ASCP), S.B.B.
Director, Medical Laboratory Technician and
Phlebotomy Programs, Montgomery County
Community College, Blue Bell, Pennsylvania
*Introduction to Phlebotomy; Equipment; Proper
Procedures for Venipuncture; Special Collection
Procedures; Complications of Phlebotomy;
Interpersonal Communication and Professionalism*

Dorothy Pfender, B.A., M.T.(ASCP), B.B.
Instructor, Montgomery County Community College,
Blue Bell, Pennsylvania
Phlebotomy Unit Management

Mary E. Paranto, M.S., M.T.(ASCP), S.B.B.
Instructor and Clinical Coordinator, Program in Medical Technology, Thomas Jefferson University, College of Allied Health Sciences, Philadelphia, Pennsylvania
Quality Assurance

Shirley E. Greening, M.S., J.D., C.F.I.A.C.
Chairman and Associate Professor, Department of Laboratory Sciences; Program Director, Cytotechnology and Cytogenetic Technology; and Health Policy Coordinator, College of Allied Health Sciences, Thomas Jefferson University, Philadelphia, Pennsylvania
Medicolegal Issues and Health Law Procedures

Preface

Procedures in Phlebotomy is intended for students of phlebotomy. These students may be just entering the field, or they may have been practicing the art of blood collection for many years. Whoever wishes to remain abreast of this rapidly changing and expanding field will find this book useful.

Procedures in Phlebotomy is divided into two sections, the first dealing with those topics directly related to blood collection, including an introduction to phlebotomy, with a brief history of the practice and a review of anatomy and physiology. Also in this section is a chapter dedicated to infectious diseases and their prevention, with special attention to Occupational Safety and Health Administration regulations. Most of this section is dedicated to a discussion of the equipment, procedures, and complications of phlebotomy. Finally, for the inquisitive student, there is a special chapter discussing small mammal venipuncture.

The second section covers professional topics such as quality assurance, interpersonal communication, and management issues and topics. This section also contains a chapter dedicated to medico-legal issues with a discussion on Clinical Laboratory Improvement Act of 1988 as it directly applies to phlebotomy.

The reader will find boldfaced terms that are defined in the glossary. Additionally, there are review questions at the end of each chapter to test the reader's comprehension, with answers provided at the back of the book. Of special interest is a 100-item review examination to aid individuals who are preparing for national certification examinations. Finally, a quick reference chart matching the color code of blood collection tubes used for commonly ordered tests is included at the front of the book.

Acknowledgments

I would like to acknowledge the efforts of several people: Linda Raichle, who was instrumental in bringing Saunders and me together; the various contributors who found time in their busy schedules to assist in the preparation of this book; Shari Center, the photographer; the people at W. B. Saunders — Selma Ozmat, Rosanne Hallowell, and Scott Weaver; Linda Pileggi; and finally, Laurene Mrusko, M.T.(ASCP), who provided invaluable contributions to the content and questions of several chapters. Without the assistance of those mentioned above and several whom I have probably forgotten, this book would never have come to fruition.

Contents

chapter **Three**

Infectious Diseases and Their Prevention................. 41
Georganne K. Buescher

chapter **Four**

Equipment...........................59
John C. Flynn, Jr.

chapter **Five**

Proper Procedures for Venipuncture............................71
John C. Flynn, Jr.

chapter **Six**

Special Collection Procedures........ 87
John C. Flynn, Jr.

chapter **Seven**

Complications of Phlebotomy....... 105
John C. Flynn, Jr.

chapter **Eight**

Animal Phlebotomy................ 117
Beth V. Dronson

part **Two** Professional Issues 133

chapter **Nine**

Interpersonal Communication and Professionalism.......................135
John C. Flynn, Jr.

chapter **Ten**

Phlebotomy Unit Management......147
Dorothy Pfender

chapter **Eleven**

Quality Assurance...................161
Mary E. Paranto

chapter **Twelve**

Medicolegal Issues and Health Law Procedures..........................179
Shirley E. Greening

EVACUATED TUBE CHARACTERISTICS

Stopper Color	Principal Anticoagulant/ Additive	Mode of Action	Common Tests
Red 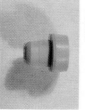	None	N/A	Cell-blood typing
	Clot activator and gel separator	Enhances clot formation	Serum blood group antibody testing
			Alkaline phosphatase
			Amylase
			Blood urea nitrogen (BUN)
			Creatine phosphokinase (CPK)
			Calcium
			Cholesterol
Speckled			Compatibility testing
			Drug monitoring
			Glucose
			High density lipoprotein (HDL)
			Human immunodeficiency virus (HIV)
Gold (Hemoguard)			Iron profile
			Low density lipoprotein (LDL)
			Liver enzymes
			Potassium
			Protein
			Rapid plasma reagin (RPR)
			Sodium
			Triglycerides
Lavender	Ethylenediaminetetraacetic acid (EDTA)	Binds calcium	Complete blood count (CBC)
			Erythrocyte sedimentation rate (ESR)
			Hemoglobin electrophoresis
			Platelet count
			Reticulocyte count
			Sickle cell screen
			White blood cell differential

Color		Additive	Action	Tests
Blue		Sodium citrate	Binds calcium	Activated partial thromboplastin time (aPTT) Individual coagulation factor studies Fibrin degradation products (FDP) Fibrinogen Prothrombin time (PT)
Green		Heparin	Inactivates thrombin and thromboplastin	Ammonia Chromosome screening Lupus erythematosus cell/preparation HLA typing
Gray		Potassium oxalate/sodium fluoride	Binds calcium Inhibits glycolysis	Glucose
Dark or royal blue		Heparin	Inactivates thrombin and thromboplastin	Trace metals, e.g., lead

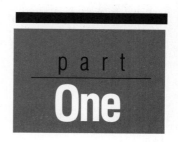

part

One

The Practice of Phlebotomy

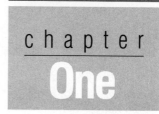
Introduction to Phlebotomy

John C. Flynn, Jr.

History
Current Phlebotomy Practice
Professional Recognition

HISTORY

"Bleed in the acute affections, if the disease appear strong, and the patients be in the vigor of life, and if they have strength." These were the thoughts of Hippocrates, recorded nearly 25 centuries ago, regarding the usefulness of **phlebotomy.** He proposed that phlebotomy be used as a treatment for acute disease conditions.

Later, during the eleventh century, when the first school of medicine was founded in Salerno in present-day Italy, "blood letting" was still a popular curative. In fact, well into modern times (that is, the seventeenth and eighteenth centuries), phlebotomy was used as a treatment for diseases ranging from mental illness to fever to convulsions (Fig. 1–1). However, as the practice of medicine and the understanding of the human body progressed, phlebotomy as a routine treatment fell into disuse.

CURRENT PHLEBOTOMY PRACTICE

Today, phlebotomy, although no longer considered a curative, is a necessary aid in the diagnosis and treatment of disease. In ancient times, witch doctors, barbers, and, later, physicians performed phlebotomies

3

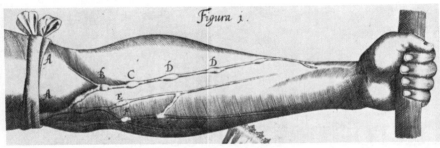

figure **1-1**   Drawing depicting the location of veins in the arm originally published in 1628. (From Harvey W: Exercitato anatomica de mortu codis et sanguinis in animalibus. Frankfurt, 1628. Courtesy of the Wellcome Institute Library, London.)

(Fig. 1-2), but in modern times trained professionals perform this vital function. These professionals, who traditionally were trained on the job, are increasingly being trained in formal programs and becoming certified by national certifying agencies (Table 1-1).

With the growth of modern medicine and the increasingly wide range of diagnostic and screening tests available, the role of the phlebotomist has become increasingly important and complex. No longer is it a matter of simply collecting a blood specimen; the modern phlebotomist must also be aware of the type of test requested, any medications the patient is taking that may interfere with the testing, the importance of the timing of the blood collection, and the effect of the patient's diet.

The modern phlebotomist may also be called on to perform other functions such as measuring bleeding times, collecting donor blood, performing therapeutic phlebotomies and bedside testing, and preparing specimens. Phlebotomists today must communicate and interact with the entire laboratory team (Fig. 1-3A). They must be familiar with both routine and special specimen requirements, including collection and transportation procedures for each section of the laboratory.

Additionally, phlebotomists must also interact and communicate with the entire health care team as well as with patients' families (Fig.

table **1-1**   PHLEBOTOMY CERTIFYING AGENCIES

American Society of Clinical Pathologists (ASCP)
American Society of Phlebotomy Technicians (ASPT)
National Certification Agency for Medical Laboratory Personnel (NCAMLP)
National Phlebotomy Association (NPA)

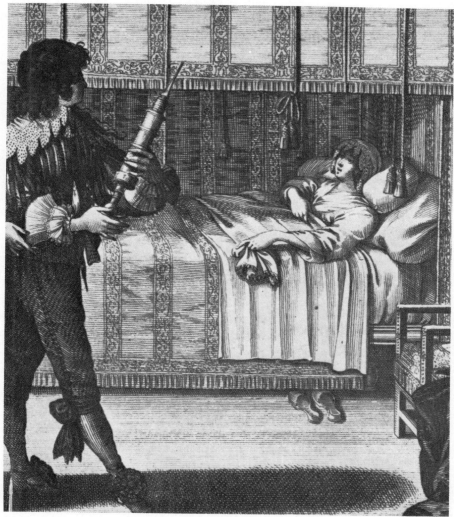

figure **1-2**   Abraham Bosse's *The Physician's Visit*. (Reproduced by Courtesy of the Trustees of the British Museum, London.)

1–3*B*). This means they must be able to "speak the language" of medicine and communicate professionally, both in writing and orally.

Furthermore, phlebotomists are not confined to working exclusively in a hospital setting. They may work in physician office laboratories, blood collection centers such as those conducted by the American Red Cross, research institutes, or veterinary offices.

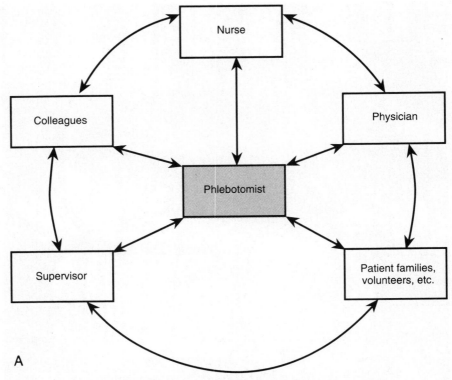

figure **1-3**   *A*, A phlebotomist's hospital communication network.

PROFESSIONAL RECOGNITION

Figure 1-4 illustrates the organizational structure of modern laboratories, with the position of the phlebotomist highlighted; it can be seen that phlebotomists are an integral part of every laboratory section and play a vital role in the health maintenance team. This partially explains the increasing number of phlebotomy training programs and the increasing number of phlebotomists becoming certified. Currently there are more than 40 approved phlebotomy programs in the United States, with more than 4000 phlebotomists certified. As has been shown in Table 1-1, there are several different accrediting agencies that certify phlebotomists, and although the examination fees and frequency of examination administration may vary, the underlying goal of all such programs is the same: to assure employers that the phlebotomists they are hiring meet a minimally acceptable standard of practice.

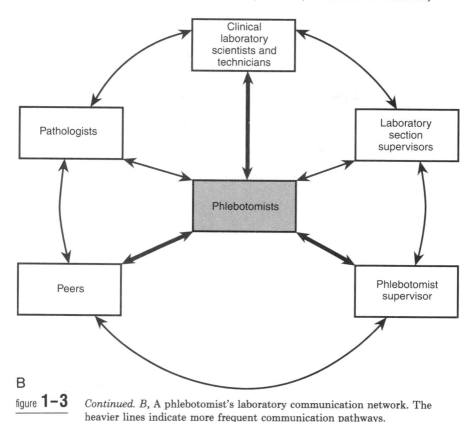

figure **1-3** *Continued. B*, A phlebotomist's laboratory communication network. The heavier lines indicate more frequent communication pathways.

Finally, all professionals should adhere to a code of conduct or a code of ethics. Early physicians followed the Hippocratic oath, and although there is no specific oath or code for phlebotomists, there is one for the field of medical technology, to which phlebotomists belong. This code is endorsed by the American Society for Medical Technology:

> Being fully cognizant of my responsibilities in the practice of Medical Technology, I affirm my willingness to discharge my duties with accuracy, thoughtfulness and care.
>
> Realizing that the knowledge obtained concerning patients in the course of my work must be treated as confidential, I hold inviolate the confidence placed in me by patients and physicians.
>
> Recognizing that my integrity and that of my profession must be pledged to the absolute reliability on my work, I will conduct myself at all times in a manner appropriate to the dignity of my profession.

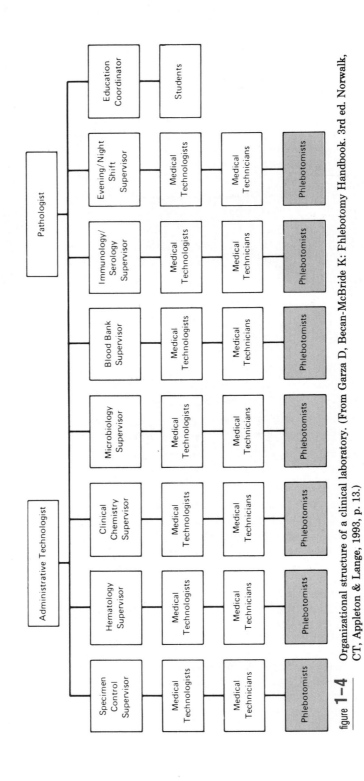

figure **1–4** Organizational structure of a clinical laboratory. (From Garza D, Becan-McBride K: Phlebotomy Handbook. 3rd ed. Norwalk, CT, Appleton & Lange, 1993, p. 13.)

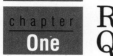

Review Questions

1. Phlebotomy is a necessary aid in the _____ and _____ of disease.
2. Before formal phlebotomy training programs existed, phlebotomists were trained _____.
3. Name some places other than hospitals that may employ phlebotomists.
4. What is the purpose of certification for phlebotomists?
5. A code of conduct that can apply to phlebotomists is published by the _____.

Bibliography

Castiglioni A. A History of Medicine. New York, Jason Aronson, 1969.
Haggard HW. Devils, Drugs, and Doctors. New York, Harper and Brothers, 1929.
Hippocrates. The Theory and Practice of Medicine. New York, Philosophical Library, 1964.
Inglis B. A History of Medicine. Cleveland, The World Publishing Company, 1965.

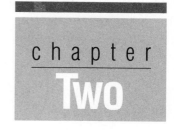

chapter

Two

Anatomy and Physiology

Barbara Janson Cohen

The human body can be studied at many levels, from the level of simple, inorganic chemicals to the level of the entire organism. Following a pattern of increasing complexity (Fig. 2–1), it can be seen that the cell is the smallest unit of life. Each cell possesses all of the qualities of life (i.e., responsiveness to the environment and the capacity for metabolism, growth, and reproduction). All of the work that goes on in the body results from the activities of individual cells; cells are the building blocks of tissues, which are groups of similar cells working together for the same

11

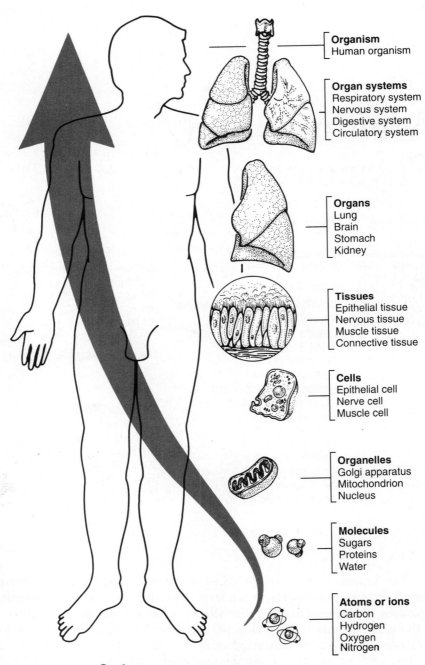

Organism
Human organism

Organ systems
Respiratory system
Nervous system
Digestive system
Circulatory system

Organs
Lung
Brain
Stomach
Kidney

Tissues
Epithelial tissue
Nervous tissue
Muscle tissue
Connective tissue

Cells
Epithelial cell
Nerve cell
Muscle cell

Organelles
Golgi apparatus
Mitochondrion
Nucleus

Molecules
Sugars
Proteins
Water

Atoms or ions
Carbon
Hydrogen
Oxygen
Nitrogen

figure **2-1**   Levels of organization of the human body.

purpose. The study of cells is known as *cytology,* and the study of tissues is *histology.*

TISSUES

There are four basic tissue types in the body:

1. *Epithelial tissue,* which is composed of simple cells that cover body structures, line organs and cavities, and form membranes. Epithelial cells are also the secreting cells of glands.

2. *Connective tissue,* which binds, supports, and protects organs and forms the structural tissues of the body such as cartilage and bone.

3. *Muscle tissue,* which moves the skeleton and forms the walls of internal organs such as the heart, digestive organs, and blood vessels.

4. *Nervous tissue,* which consists of highly specialized cells that transmit electrical signals throughout the body.

Each organ in the body is a complex of different tissues. Even bone, which consists mainly of connective tissue, is supplied with blood vessels and nerves. The heart, made mostly of cardiac muscle, contains other tissues as well.

ORGAN SYSTEMS

Currently, study of the anatomy (structure) and physiology (function) of the body generally centers on study of the body systems. A *system* is defined as a group of organs working together to perform related functions. Many medical specialties concentrate on one body system; for instance, neurology is the study of the nervous system, gastroenterology is the study of the digestive system, and orthopedics is the study of the musculoskeletal system. Usually, the organs in the system are anatomically connected, but in some cases, as with the endocrine system of hormone-secreting glands, the tissues are widely distributed. The so-called "immune system" involves components of other systems, including the cardiovascular and lymphatic systems.

Of course, all body systems work together at all times and constantly interact to maintain a state of internal balance known as *homeostasis.* A disturbance in any organ or system may affect other systems of the body.

In this chapter we will briefly discuss each of the organ systems, with special emphasis on the circulatory system.

DESCRIPTIONS OF BODY SYSTEMS

In the following brief descriptions, body systems are grouped according to their main functions. We begin with the integumentary system.

The Integumentary System

The integumentary system consists of the skin and associated structures (Fig. 2–2). The outermost layer of the skin is the *epidermis*. Under this is the true skin, or *dermis*, which rests on the *subcutaneous layer*, a layer composed of connective tissue and adipose (fat) tissue. The skin is well supplied with blood vessels and with a variety of receptors for senses such as touch, pressure, pain, and temperature. Also associated with the skin are hair follicles, nails, sweat glands, and sebaceous glands, which secrete an oily lubricant called *sebum*. The integumentary system protects underlying tissues, prevents dehydration, keeps out foreign organisms, and is used to regulate body temperature. The skin, hair, and nails provide easily observed signs of an individual's state of health; their examination is useful in diagnosis.

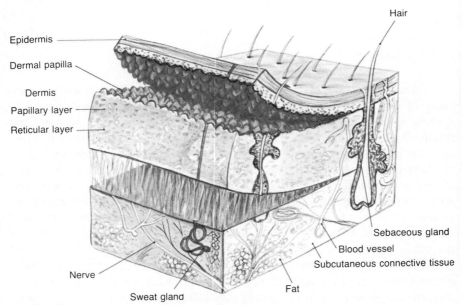

figure **2–2**   Cross section of the skin. (From Dienhart CM. Basic Human Anatomy and Physiology. 3rd ed. Philadelphia, PA, WB Saunders, 1979, p. 26.)

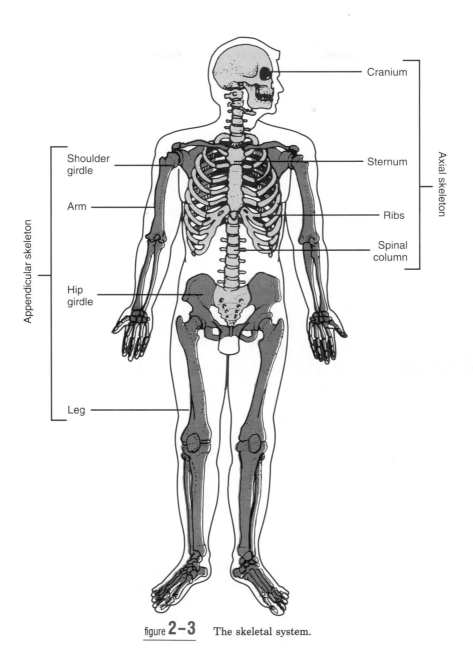

figure **2-3**   The skeletal system.

Systems Needed for Movement and Support

THE SKELETAL SYSTEM

The bones of the skeleton (Fig. 2–3) are divided into an *axial* portion, consisting of the cranium, spinal column, ribs, and sternum, and an *appendicular* portion, consisting of the shoulder girdle, the hip girdle, and the bones of the arms and legs. The skeleton gives the body structure, protects vital organs, and works with the muscular system to produce movement at the joints. Blood cells are produced within the red marrow of the bones.

THE MUSCULAR SYSTEM

There are three types of muscle tissue: **smooth (visceral) muscle,** which makes up the walls of hollow organs and the blood vessels; **cardiac muscle,** which makes up the heart; and **skeletal (striated) muscle,** which is attached to the bones. The term *muscular system* refers to the last of these, the more than 700 muscles that move the skeleton (Fig. 2–4). The main property of muscle tissue is the ability to contract in response to stimulation by the nervous system. To function, muscles need

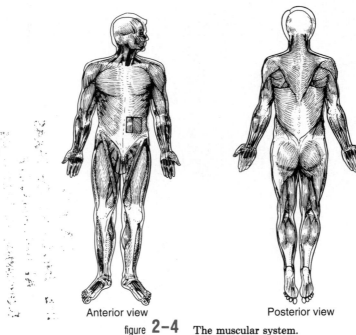

Anterior view   Posterior view

figure **2–4**   The muscular system.

a source of energy, such as glucose; oxygen to release the energy from the nutrient; and calcium for the interactions of contractile filaments within the muscle cells. Muscles can function for a brief period without oxygen, but when they do, they accumulate **lactic acid,** which soon causes muscle fatigue. As they work, muscles generate heat. For example, shivering on a cold day boosts the energy output of the skeletal muscles to warm the body.

Systems That Control and Coordinate Activities

THE NERVOUS SYSTEM

The nervous system (Fig. 2–5) is divided for study into a *central nervous system* (CNS), consisting of the brain and spinal cord, and a *peripheral nervous system* (PNS), comprising all nervous tissue outside of the CNS, including the cranial and spinal nerves that connect with the brain and spinal cord and the receptors, which respond to changes in the

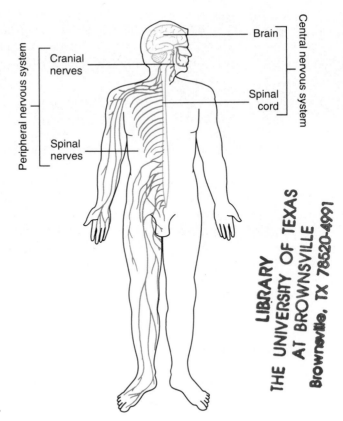

figure **2–5**

The nervous system.

internal and external environments. The purpose of the nervous system is to detect such changes, known as *stimuli,* and to coordinate an appropriate response. The nervous system works by transmitting electrical signals along nerve cells, or *neurons.* It also employs chemicals, called *neurotransmitters,* to carry a stimulus across the junctions between nerve cells, contact points known as *synapses.* Information is coordinated and interpreted within the CNS, which then directs a suitable response by a muscle or a gland.

A functional subdivision of the nervous system is the *autonomic nervous system,* which controls involuntary (unconscious) behavior. It consists of two portions: the *sympathetic system,* which stimulates an alarm response ("fight-or-flight" response), and the *parasympathetic system,* which restores balance and stimulates maintenance systems such as the digestive and urinary systems.

THE SENSORY SYSTEM

The sensory system is a component of the nervous system and contains specialized cells that can detect stimuli. These cells, or *receptors,* may be widely distributed throughout the body or localized in special sense organs. The latter include the ear (hearing and equilibrium), the eye (vision), the tongue (taste), and the nose (smell). General receptors detect pain, temperature, touch, pressure, and body position.

THE ENDOCRINE SYSTEM

The endocrine system (Fig. 2–6) consists of glands that secrete substances that affect other cells. These substances, called **hormones,** are released into the bloodstream to be carried to the target cells. They exert a wide range of effects on growth, metabolism, reproduction, and behavior. Examples of hormones include steroid hormones secreted by the adrenal glands and the sex glands, insulin secreted by the pancreas, thyroid hormone, and growth hormone secreted by the pituitary gland. The *pituitary* gland, which secretes a number of hormones that regulate other endocrine glands, is actually controlled by the hypothalamus, a region of the brain just above it. Although hormone-secreting glands are collectively referred to as the endocrine system, there are other organs that release hormones. These include the kidneys, stomach, intestine, and heart.

Systems That Transport Materials

THE CARDIOVASCULAR SYSTEM

As the name suggests, the cardiovascular system (Fig. 2–7) consists of the heart and blood vessels. Together these form a closed circuit for

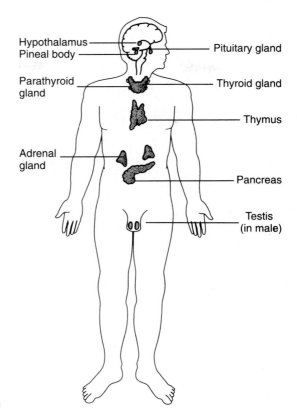

Hypothalamus

Pineal body

Parathyroid gland

Adrenal gland

Pituitary gland

Thyroid gland

Thymus

Pancreas

Testis (in male)

figure **2-6**

The endocrine system.

carrying blood to and from the tissues. Blood brings nutrients and oxygen to the cells and carries away metabolic wastes and carbon dioxide. The blood also carries hormones, antibodies, and enzymes. As it circulates, the blood distributes body heat, which is generated largely by muscles and glands. This system is of major interest to phlebotomists and will be discussed in greater detail later.

THE LYMPHATIC SYSTEM

The lymphatic system (Fig. 2–8) works with the cardiovascular system to provide effective circulation. Unlike the blood vessels, which form a closed circuit, the lymphatic vessels form a one-way system that drains excess fluids and proteins from the tissues and returns them to the subclavian veins near the heart. The *thoracic duct* drains the lower portion and the upper left half of the body and empties into the left subclavian vein; the *right lymphatic duct* drains the upper right half of the body and empties into the right subclavian vein. The fluid that circulates in the lymphatic system is called **lymph.**

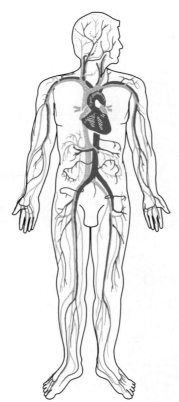

figure **2-7**

The cardiovascular system.

The lymphatic system has some other functions as well. It collects digested fats through special capillaries, called *lacteals,* in the villi of the small intestine. These nutrients are added to the general circulation when the lymph joins the blood.

Finally, the lymphatic system is considered to be part of the immune system. Lymphatic tissues help to filter blood and other body fluids, and cells active in immunity (lymphocytes) are sheltered and stimulated within organs of the lymphatic system. Lymphatic organs include the lymph nodes, which are located throughout the body; the spleen; the thymus gland; the tonsils; and the appendix.

Systems Involved in Energy Metabolism

THE RESPIRATORY SYSTEM

The function of the respiratory system (Fig. 2-9) is to supply the body with **oxygen** needed for metabolism of food. Air is drawn into the

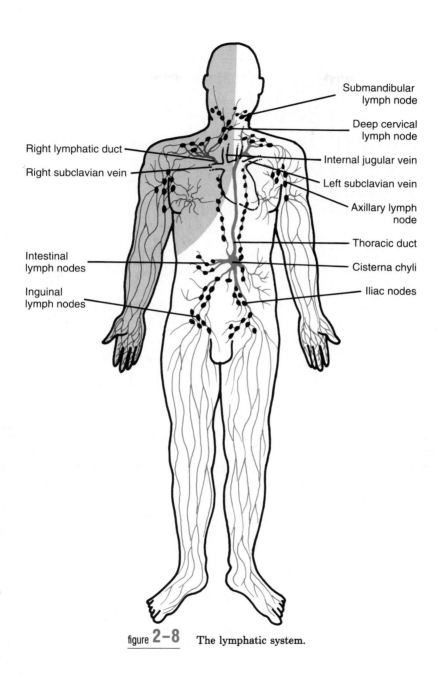

figure **2-8**   The lymphatic system.

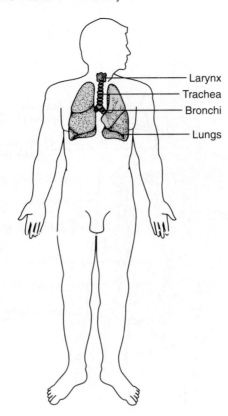

Larynx
Trachea
Bronchi
Lungs

figure **2-9**

The respiratory system.

lungs as the diaphragm flattens and the rib cage is elevated to enlarge the chest cavity. In traveling toward the lungs, air passes through the nose, throat (pharnyx), larnyx (voicebox), trachea (windpipe), bronchi, and the smaller bronchioles. Once the air reaches the **alveoli,** the tiny air sacs at the ends of the respiratory passageways, oxygen is absorbed into the bloodstream to be transported to the cells.

The lungs also serve to eliminate **carbon dioxide,** the gaseous waste product of metabolism. This activity affects the relative acidity (pH) of body fluids.

THE DIGESTIVE SYSTEM

For nutrients to be of use, they must be in a form small enough to pass through the membrane that surrounds each cell. It is the digestive system (Fig. 2–10) that receives food and breaks it down into its useful components. As food is moved through the digestive tract by wavelike contractions known as *peristalsis,* it is mixed with digestive juices that split large molecules into smaller ones. Most of these secretions are

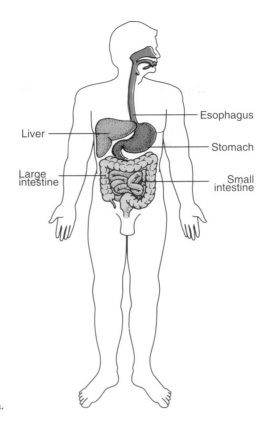

Liver

Large
intestine

Esophagus

Stomach

Small
intestine

figure **2-10**

The digestive system.

enzymes, chemicals that catalyze metabolic reactions in the body. Most digestion occurs in the small intestine under the effects of enzymes secreted by the small intestine, along with additional substances contributed by the liver and pancreas. The liver produces bile, which emulsifies fats, and the pancreas contributes a mixture of digestive enzymes. Before delivery to the small intestine, bile is stored in the gallbladder, a small sac under the liver.

The products of digestion are also absorbed into the circulation in the small intestine. The transfer occurs through the villi, tiny fingerlike projections in the lining of the organ that contain blood capillaries and lacteals of the lymphatic system. The building blocks of proteins and carbohydrates are absorbed directly into the bloodstream; the building blocks of fats enter the lymphatic system. The final steps in digestion are the storage of undigested waste and its elimination from the body by the large intestine.

The nutrient products of digestion are used by cells to generate energy and manufacture needed substances. All of the chemical reactions that occur within the body are collectively referred to as **metabolism.** Reactions in which complex substances are broken down into smaller components constitute *catabolism;* the building of these small molecules into larger products is termed *anabolism.*

THE URINARY SYSTEM

The urinary system (Fig. 2–11) consists of the two kidneys; the paired ureters that carry urine from the kidneys; the bladder, where urine is stored until elimination; and the single urethra, which carries urine out of the body. In females, the urinary system is entirely separated from the reproductive system. In males, the urethra carries both urine and semen, and the two systems are sometimes studied together as the *urogenital system.* The formation of urine is accomplished by the kidneys. Here, microscopic working units, called *nephrons,* filter the blood and selectively remove substances for inclusion in the urine. Although much material leaves the blood initially, most is returned to the circulation by the

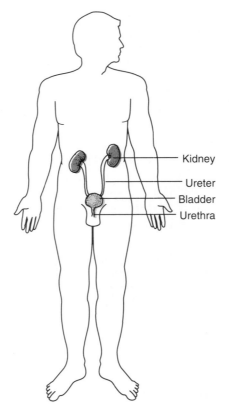

Kidney

Ureter

Bladder

Urethra

figure **2–11**

The urinary system.

process of reabsorption. The kidneys adjust the final product to eliminate waste such as urea and toxins, and to balance the water, electrolytes (dissolved salts), and pH (acidity) of body fluids.

In addition to the above activities, the kidneys also secrete the enzyme *renin,* which acts to increase blood pressure when released into the bloodstream and the hormone *erythropoietin,* which stimulates the production of red blood cells in the bone marrow.

The Reproductive System

The reproductive glands, or **gonads,** are responsible for producing the sex cells, also known as *gametes.* In the male the gonads are the *testes,* which produce sperm cells, or spermatozoa; in the female, they are the *ovaries,* which produce egg cells, or ova (Fig. 2–12). A second function of the gonads is to produce hormones. These substances are active in the reproductive process and also have generalized effects on the body, such as promoting the secondary sex characteristics that are associated with gender. In both males and females, reproductive activity is initiated by hormones released from the pituitary gland. As previously noted, the pituitary gland is actually controlled by the hypothalamus of the brain.

From puberty on, sperm cells are generated continuously in the male under the effects of testosterone and other male hormones. The cells are transported out of the body through a series of ducts, terminating with the urethra, which passes through the penis. Several glands — the seminal vesicles, prostate, and bulbourethral glands — contribute secretions that

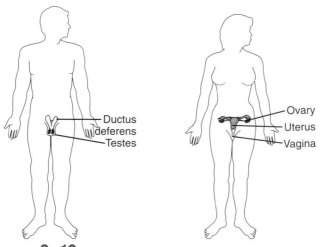

figure **2–12**   The male and female reproductive systems.

form semen, the fluid that transports, protects, and nourishes the sperm cells.

Gamete formation in the female is cyclic. Each month several eggs ripen under the effects of hormones from the pituitary gland. About midway in the menstrual cycle, one egg is released, an event termed *ovulation*. If the egg is fertilized, forming a zygote, it will attach to the wall of the uterus and begin development, first as an embryo and then, after the second month, as a fetus. In the event that the egg is not fertilized, hormone levels decline, and menstrual flow begins. During the course of the menstrual cycle, the ovaries produce first estrogen and then progesterone, both of which stimulate development of the endometrium, the lining of the uterus. These hormones feed back to inhibit the secretion of hormones from the pituitary, thus creating a cyclic pattern of activity.

THE CARDIOVASCULAR SYSTEM

The Heart

STRUCTURE

The heart (Fig. 2–13) is a muscular organ responsible for the continuous pumping of blood through the vascular system. It is divided by a septum (wall) into right and left sides. The right side pumps blood to the lungs through the pulmonary circuit; the left side pumps blood to the remainder of the body through the systemic circuit (Fig. 2–14). Because it has to push blood through a longer circuit, the left side of the heart is larger, and the myocardium (muscular wall) is thicker. The upper, blood-receiving chamber on each side is called an *atrium* (pl., atria); the lower, blood-pumping chamber on each side is called a *ventricle* (pl., ventricles). Two large vessels, the superior vena cava and the inferior vena cava, bring blood back to the right atrium from the upper and lower parts of the body. Blood is then pumped to the lungs through the pulmonary arteries and returned to the left atrium through the pulmonary veins. The largest artery, the aorta, carries blood from the left ventricle into the systemic circuit. Between the chambers on each side there is a valve that keeps blood flowing in a forward direction as the heart pumps. On the right is the tricuspid valve, so named because it has three flaps. On the left is the bicuspid, or mitral, valve. There are also valves at the entrance to the large vessels (pulmonary artery and aorta) that carry blood away from the heart. Because each flap of these valves resembles a half-moon, they are termed semilunar valves.

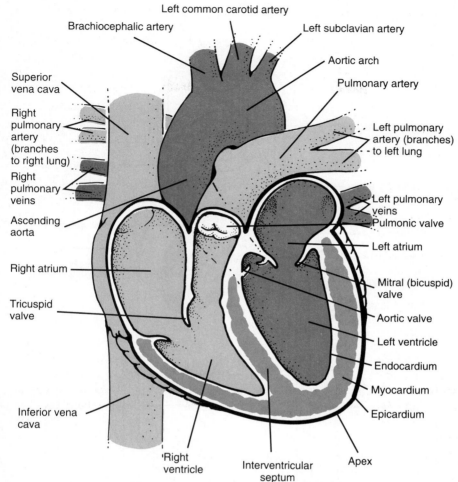

figure **2-13**   Diagram of the heart showing the chambers, valves, and direction of blood flow.

The entire heart is enclosed in a fibrous sac, the pericardium. The thin membrane that lines the chambers and covers the valve flaps is the endocardium.

HEARTBEAT

The heart is described as having intrinsic beat, which means that the heartbeat originates within the heart itself. In the upper part of the right atrium (Fig. 2–15) there is a tiny bit of nervous tissue, the sinoatrial

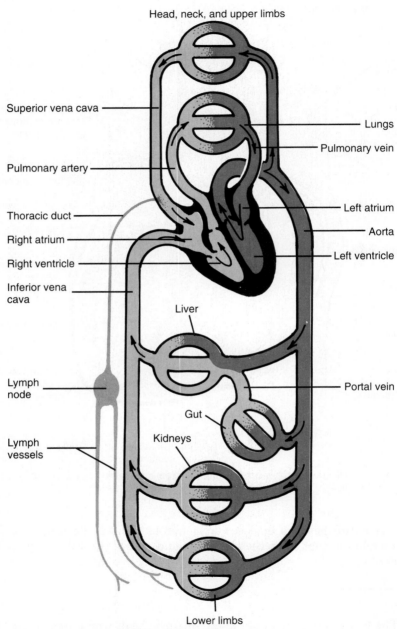

Head, neck, and upper limbs

Superior vena cava

Lungs

Pulmonary vein

Pulmonary artery

Thoracic duct

Left atrium

Aorta

Right atrium

Right ventricle

Left ventricle

Inferior vena cava

Liver

Lymph node

Portal vein

Gut

Kidneys

Lymph vessels

Lower limbs

figure **2−14**   The blood circuit.

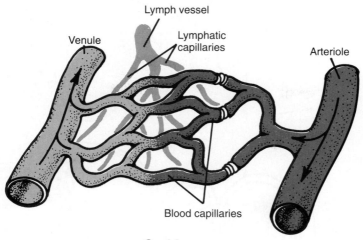

figure **2-14**   *Continued*

(SA) node, that emits an electrical impulse at a regular rate of about 72 times per minute. Because it sets the basic rate of heart contractions, the SA node is popularly called the *pacemaker*. (An artificial pacemaker is a device that provides this function for an ailing heart). From this node, the electrical impulse spreads through the atria and to the atrioventricular (AV) node in the lower part of the right atrium. It then travels through the AV bundle, which carries the impulse to the right and left bundle branches along the septum between the two ventricles. The fibers in the two branches, known as *Purkinje fibers,* then branch throughout the ventricular myocardium. This electrical activity spreads very rapidly through the heart with each beat, stimulating a contraction first of both atria and then of both ventricles. The contraction phase of the heart cycle is termed **systole** (adj., systolic), and the relaxation phase is **diastole** (adj., diastolic). The amount of blood pumped out of the left ventricle with each beat is the stroke volume. The amount ejected in 1 minute, a product of the stroke volume and heart rate, is the cardiac output. This volume averages 5 L for an adult at rest, an amount approximately equal to the total blood volume of the body.

Although the heart rate is intrinsically set, it can be influenced by a number of factors. The heart rate varies under different conditions. The autonomic nervous system acts to increase cardiac output (sympathetic division) or decrease cardiac output (parasympathetic division). Other factors that influence heart action are physical conditioning and hormones, drugs, and ions in the blood.

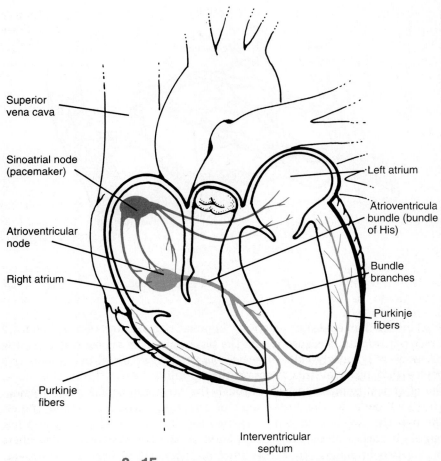

Superior
vena cava

Sinoatrial node
(pacemaker)

Atrioventricular
node

Right atrium

Purkinje
fibers

Left atrium

Atrioventricula
bundle (bundle
of His)

Bundle
branches

Purkinje
fibers

Interventricular
septum

figure **2 – 15**   The conduction system of the heart.

The Blood Vessels

Barring injury, blood circulates at all times within blood vessels. These vessels, along with the heart, form a closed circuit that transports blood to all parts of the body. The vessels that carry blood away from the heart are the *arteries* (Fig. 2–16A). The arteries and their smaller counterparts, the *arterioles,* generally carry blood that is high in oxygen. The only exceptions to this rule are the pulmonary arteries, which carry blood from the right side of the heart to the lungs for oxygenation, and the umbilical arteries in the fetus, which carry blood to the placenta for the same purpose. Blood flows from the arterial system into the smallest of the vessels, the *capillaries;* through the walls of the capillaries, exchanges take place between the bloodstream and the tissues. Blood then flows back to the heart, first in small vessels called *venules* and then in larger versions of these vessels, the *veins* (Fig. 2–16*B*). Most veins carry blood that is lower in oxygen than that in the arteries, except for the pulmonary and umbilical veins.

STRUCTURE

Blood vessels differ somewhat in structure (Fig. 2–17). The arteries have a relatively thick wall and a small central opening (lumen). The vessel wall is composed of smooth muscle controlled by the autonomic (involuntary) nervous system. The larger arteries also contain elastic tissue that maintains the shape of the vessels and puts pressure on the blood within them. The lining of the vessels is a thin, smooth layer of epithelial tissue known as *endothelium.*

The veins have the same layers, but a thinner wall with less elastic tissue. Thus veins expand more when filled with blood and carry blood under lower pressure. Valves along the path of the veins keep blood flowing in a forward direction toward the heart. The squeezing of the veins by skeletal muscles during movement also helps to drive blood back to the heart. Still, the veins are considered to be a reservoir for the blood, as more of the total blood volume is in the venous system at any one time than in the arterial system.

The capillaries (Fig. 2–18), the tiniest of the vessels, are microscopic in size. Their walls consist of only the innermost layer of vascular tissue, the very thin endothelium, which is composed of a single layer of flat epithelial cells. It is through and between the cells of the capillary walls that substances move back and forth between the blood and the tissues. The blood delivers oxygen and nutrients, as well as hormones, minerals, enzymes, and other special substances, to the cells. As it leaves the capillary beds, the blood picks up cellular secretions, carbon dioxide, urea, and other waste products of metabolism.

PULSE AND BLOOD PRESSURE

With each beat of the heart, a wave of increased pressure is sent through the vessels. This wave, or *pulse,* can be felt at arteries close to the surface of the body. Vessels commonly used for measuring the pulse rate are the radial artery at the inner surface of the wrist, thumb side; the carotid artery in the neck; and the dorsalis pedis on the top of the foot.

Blood pressure is the force of the blood against the walls of the blood

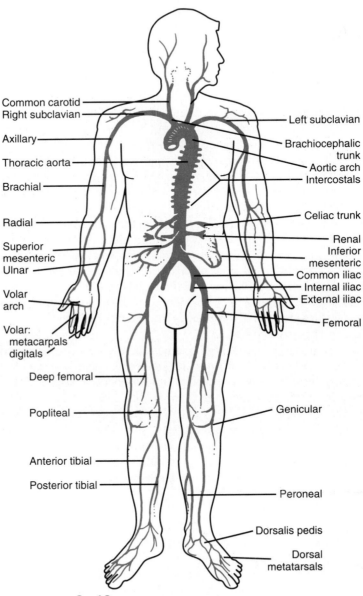

figure **2-16**   Blood vessels. *A,* The major arteries.

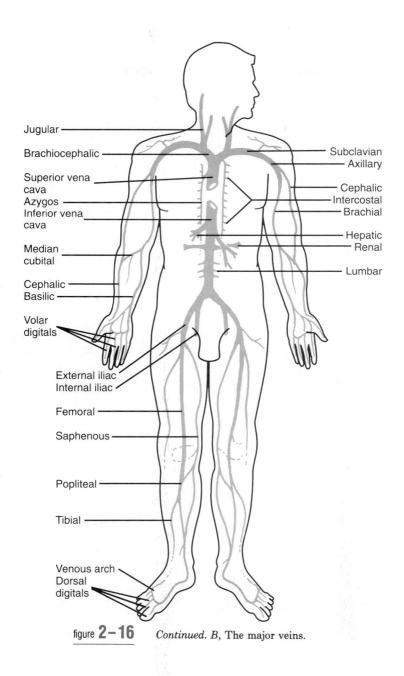

Jugular

Brachiocephalic

Superior vena cava

Azygos

Inferior vena cava

Median cubital

Cephalic

Basilic

Volar digitals

External iliac

Internal iliac

Femoral

Saphenous

Popliteal

Tibial

Venous arch

Dorsal digitals

Subclavian

Axillary

Cephalic

Intercostal

Brachial

Hepatic

Renal

Lumbar

figure **2-16**   *Continued. B,* The major veins.

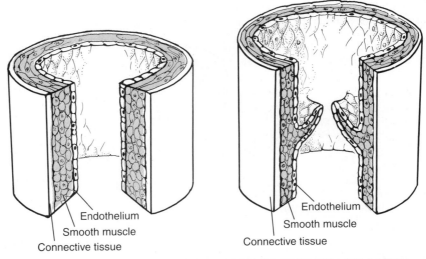

CROSS-SECTION OF AN ARTERY   CROSS-SECTION OF A VEIN

figure **2–17**   Structure of blood vessels.

vessels. It is generally measured in the brachial artery of the upper arm using a **sphygmomanometer,** or a blood pressure cuff. Pressure is measured both when the heart is contracting (systole) and when it is relaxing (diastole) and is reported as the systolic pressure over the diastolic pressure (e.g., 120/80). There are many factors that can affect blood pressure,

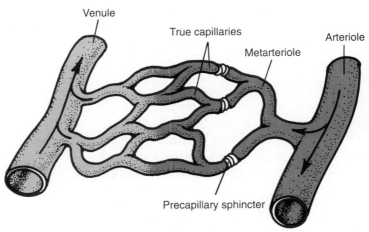

figure **2–18**   Capillary network connecting an arteriole with a venule.

which is why this measurement is such a valuable diagnostic tool. These factors include the following:

1. Cardiac output
2. Total blood volume in the system
3. Thickness (viscosity) of the blood
4. Elasticity of the blood vessels
5. Diameter of the blood vessels
6. Hormones

The diameter of the blood vessels is altered by contraction and relaxation of smooth muscle in the walls of the vessels. The involuntary nervous system governs these changes, which are known as *vasoconstriction* (narrowing) and *vasodilation* (widening). These movements control blood pressure in the vessels and the distribution of blood to various parts of the body.

The state in which blood pressure is abnormally high is termed **hypertension.** A number of disorders can result in hypertension, but a common cause is oversecretion of the enzyme renin from the kidneys. This enzyme initiates a series of steps that results in an elevation of blood pressure.

The Blood

Whole blood consists of a liquid, known as *plasma,* and blood cells. Plasma, which constitutes about 55% of the blood, contains mostly water along with nutrients, gases, waste materials, electrolytes (salts), clotting factors, and special substances such as antibodies and hormones. The remaining 45% of the blood, the blood cells, includes the red blood cells, white blood cells, and platelets (Fig. 2–19). All blood cells are manufactured in the red bone marrow, although some white blood cells can multiply in lymphatic tissue as well.

BLOOD CELLS

Red blood cells, or *erythrocytes,* number about 5 million per cubic millimeter (microliter) of blood. Their job is to carry oxygen around in the bloodstream bound to the pigment **hemoglobin.** In the tissues, the oxygen that is picked up in the lungs is released to the cells for metabolic activities. Red cells live for about 120 days before they wear out and must be replaced.

White blood cells number about 5000 to 10,000 per cubic millimeter of blood. These cells, also called *leukocytes,* are classified according to the presence or absence of granules in the cytoplasm and the staining properties of the cells. *Neutrophils,* the most common of the granular leukocytes, are phagocytes—that is, they ingest foreign organisms and materials. These cells, technically known as polymorphonuclear leukocytes, are commonly referred to as *polys, polymorphs, segs,* or *PMNs*

Agranular leukocytes are active in immunity. The *monocytes* are agranular phagocytic cells that function in destroying foreign organisms. The *lymphocytes,* which can live and multiply in the lymphatic system, are the major components of the immune system. *B cells* produce antibodies, and *T cells* attack foreign organisms directly.

Platelets, also called *thrombocytes,* participate in blood clotting. When vessels are damaged, the platelets release factors that are needed for the clotting reactions. Because platelets are not whole cells but fragments of larger cells, the blood cells are sometimes referred to as *formed elements.*

BLOOD CLOTTING

Blood clotting, or *coagulation,* is the final step in *hemostasis,* the prevention of blood loss. Platelets aid in this process by forming a plug to stop flow from a damaged vessel and then releasing substances that act in coagulation. More than a dozen *clotting factors* present in the blood plasma are needed for clotting to occur. The final reaction involves the conversion of a precursor into *fibrin,* which forms a meshwork, trapping cells and platelets in an insoluble clot. The fluid that remains after blood has clotted is called *serum.*

BLOOD TYPING

Often blood must be "typed" and "crossmatched" before a transfusion can be given. What does this actually mean? On their surface, blood cells have specific proteins (antigens) that vary in different individuals according to their genetic makeup. The first to be discovered, and the best known of these proteins, comprise a group known as the *ABO system* (Fig. 2–20). An individual may have the A antigen only (type A), the B antigen only (type B), both antigens (type AB), or neither antigen (type O). Each person has antibodies to whichever antigen is absent from his or her own blood. If blood with a foreign antigen is administered, the plasma of the recipient will react with the donor cells, causing an adverse response known as a *transfusion reaction.* Blood can be tested for the various surface antigens using antiserum prepared against each. The cells will clump, or agglutinate, in the presence of the corresponding antibody.

It is always best to give blood of a matching type. However, in an emergency, persons with both antigens on the surface of their cells (type

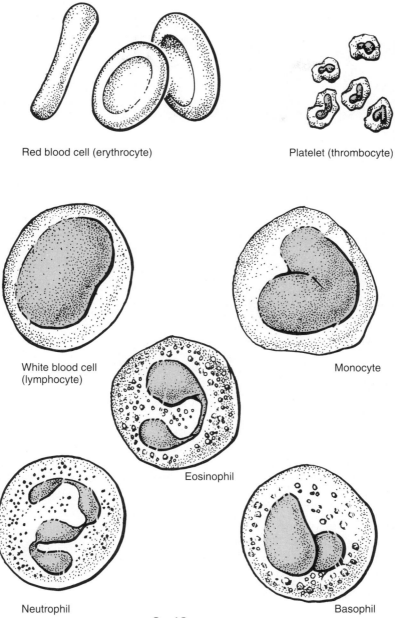

Red blood cell (erythrocyte)

Platelet (thrombocyte)

White blood cell
(lymphocyte)

Monocyte

Eosinophil

Neutrophil

Basophil

figure **2–19**   Blood cells.

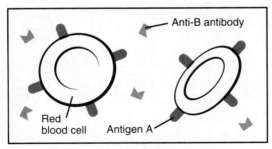

Type A blood

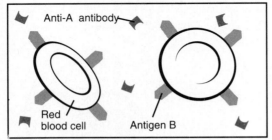

Type B blood

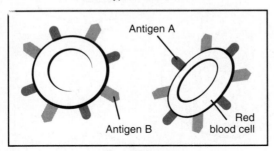

Type AB blood

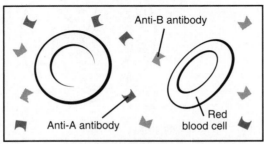

A Type O blood

figure **2–20**

Blood groups. *A*, Antigens and antibodies in the A, B, AB, and O blood groups.

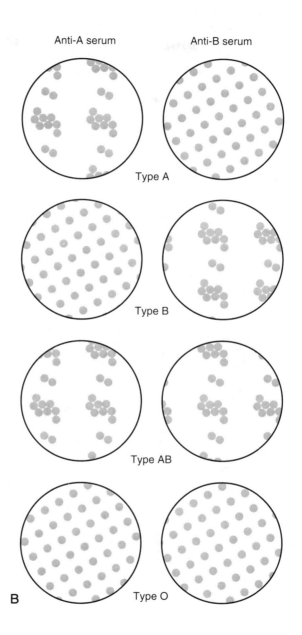

figure **2–20**

Continued. B, Blood typing.   **B**

table **2-1** THE ABO BLOOD GROUP SYSTEM

Blood Type	Antigen	Antibodies	Can Receive From	Can Donate To
A	A	Anti-B	A, O	A, AB
B	B	Anti-A	B, O	B, AB
AB	A, B	None	AB, A, B, O	AB
O	None	Anti-A, anti-B	O	O, A, B, AB

AB) can take blood of any ABO type, and persons with type O can give blood to any ABO type (Table 2–1).

Many other blood cell antigens have been discovered since the identification of the A and B antigens. One is the Rh factor, or D antigen. Individuals are designated as Rh positive (Rh+) or Rh negative (Rh−) depending on the presence or absence of the D antigen on the surface of their cells.

chapter
Two

Review Questions

1. The _____ is the smallest unit of life.
2. A group of organs working together to perform related functions is defined as a _____.
3. _____ muscle makes up the heart.
4. The _____ are responsible for producing gametes.
5. _____ aid in the coagulation process by forming a plug to stop blood flow.

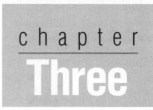

chapter
Three

Infectious Diseases and Their Prevention

Georganne K. Buescher

Numerous diseases can be transmitted by contact with an infected person or a source of contamination. Phlebotomists, as health care professionals, will be asked to take blood from **infectious** persons, and it is therefore important for them to become familiar with the infectious diseases that pose the greatest risk to them—especially those diseases that are transmitted through contact with blood. This chapter will familiarize health care workers with those infections that pose occupational risks for phlebotomists and the precautions that must be taken for protection. Many patients with transmissible, blood-borne diseases such as chronic hepatitis (hepatitis B) or the human immunodeficiency virus (HIV) infection may be asymptomatic when they are admitted to the hospital and

---

table **3-1**   ACCEPTABLE HAND WASHING TECHNIQUE

---

1. Wash hands before and after entering a patient's room.
2. Remove jewelry on hands and wrists.
3. Wet hands under running water.
4. Keep hands down and apply soap or antiseptic hand scrub.
5. Employ friction to clean all surfaces of the hands and wrists.
6. Rinse thoroughly under running water.
7. Dry hands thoroughly with paper towels.
8. Use paper towels to turn off the faucet to prevent contamination.

---

unaware that they are infected. However, the risk of transmission to the phlebotomist is extremely low if proper precautions are learned and carried out for *all* patients. Frequent, thorough hand washing (Table 3-1) is the most important preventive measure that can be taken by health care professionals.

Pathogens of all four major groups of microorganisms (bacteria, fungi, viruses, and parasites) may be carried in the blood during the course of a specific disease. Over the years, the risk of occupation-associated infections has shifted in focus from bacterial to viral infections. Today, the viruses of greatest concern to health care professionals are the hepatitis B virus (HBV) and HIV. These viruses are transmitted almost exclusively through infected blood and blood products.

VIRAL INFECTIOUS DISEASES

Viral **nosocomial** infections are an important **epidemiologic** concern for health care providers. Because of their contact with patients, phlebotomists are at risk for transmission of vaccine-preventable viral diseases. Immunization protocols for employees in health care institutions can provide safeguards against infection for personnel as well as for patients, since viruses can be transmitted from patients to staff, as well as from staff to patients.

Today there is a focus on the health care institution's responsibility to protect employees from infection. The institution must ensure that employees such as phlebotomists who are at risk for infection have been immunized properly. Laboratory screening tests are available to determine a person's immunization status for a wide range of infectious diseases, including hepatitis, measles, polio, mumps, rubella, and chickenpox.

table **3-2**   CHARACTERISTICS OF ACUTE VIRAL HEPATITIS

	Hepatitis A (HAV)	Hepatitis B (HBV)	Hepatitis C (HCV)
Epidemiology	Fecal-oral	Parenteral	Parenteral and nonparenteral
Incubation period			
(days)	15–45	40–180	15–150
Asymptomatic infection	Usual	Common	Common
Chronicity	No	Yes	Yes

Viral Hepatitis

Hepatitis is a systemic disease primarily involving the liver. There are several types of hepatitis virus infections with differing modes of transmission: hepatitis A virus (HAV), also known as infectious hepatitis or short incubation hepatitis; HBV, also known as serum hepatitis or long-incubation hepatitis; and the recently identified hepatitis C virus (HCV), which is associated with blood transfusions. All types of viral hepatitis produce an acute inflammation of the liver, which causes a clinical illness characterized by fever, nausea, vomiting, and jaundice. Table 3-2 presents a comparison of HAV, HBV, and HCV infections.

HAV is transmitted most often by the fecal-oral route. Phlebotomists may become infected by contact with a patient's feces or blood.

HCV accounts for the majority of post-transfusion cases of hepatitis in the United States. It was not until 1990, when laboratory tests for the detection of antibodies against HCV became available, that the frequency of HCV infection was recognized. Chronic liver disease is a frequent outcome of HCV infection. After infection, disease may take years to develop, and the majority of infected individuals are asymptomatic. Health care professionals with occupational exposure to blood are at increased risk of acquiring HCV infections.

HBV INFECTION

HBV infection is recognized by the Centers for Disease Control (CDC) as a major occupational hazard for health care workers. It is the most frequently reported occupation-associated infection for persons who handle blood or blood products. The risk of infection is much higher for health care professionals than for the general population, and worldwide, HBV is a leading cause of acute and chronic hepatitis, cirrhosis of the liver, and primary hepatocellular carcinoma. According to the CDC, the risk of acquiring HBV infection is dependent on the frequency of **percutaneous** exposures to blood.[2] Phlebotomists, because of the procedures that they perform, are at risk for HBV infection from needlesticks with contaminated needles.

HBV is global in its distribution. In the United States alone there are approximately 1 million carriers, about 25% of whom will go on to develop chronic active hepatitis. Chronic carriers may or may not have the typical signs and symptoms of liver disease and may not be recognized as high-risk patients (i.e., patients with infections that can be passed on to those who care for them).

The incubation period for HBV is between 50 and 180 days, with a mean onset time of 60 to 90 days after transmission.

Prevention

The risk of acquiring HBV infection from occupational exposures depends on the frequency of percutaneous or **permucosal** exposures to blood or blood products. As little as 0.0001 ml of infected **plasma** (about 1/500 of a drop—much too small to see) can transmit this disease. Therefore, the most important preventive measure to reduce the potential for HBV transmission is the use of gloves.

HBV is a vaccine-preventable disease, and therefore it is recommended that persons in the health professions complete a vaccination program during their training, before their first contact with blood.[3] Recent Federal Occupational Safety and Health Administration (OSHA) regulations require that all health care personnel at risk for exposure to HBV receive hepatitis B vaccination. The vaccines (Recombivax-HB, Engerix-B) have been shown to be safe, immunogenic, and effective in preventing HBV infection. Three inoculations are given for protection: an initial injection, a second injection 1 month later, and a third injection 6 months after the first injection. A blood test can be done to be sure protective antibodies have developed. A consistent program of vaccinations would eliminate the problem of having susceptible health care workers in hospitals.[2]

The CDC has developed guidelines for postexposure **prophylaxis** in a nonimmune individual exposed to HBV. The person should immediately receive both hepatitis B immune globulin (HBIG) and the hepatitis B vaccine. The injections should be administered simultaneously at different sites. HBIG provides immediate protection with passively acquired antibody; the active immunity produced by the vaccine develops over several weeks.

Patients with an acute HBV infection generally are not placed in strict isolation when they are hospitalized. They may remain in a regular room as long as blood and instrument precautions are strictly followed on the floor and in the laboratory.

HIV Infection

HIV is a member of the retrovirus family of RNA viruses. It is the primary **etiologic** agent of the acquired immunodeficiency syndrome (AIDS) and the AIDS-related complex. AIDS was first described in 1981, but it was not until 1983 that the causative viral agent was isolated. Today, AIDS has reached epidemic proportions worldwide, with tens of thousands of cases in the United States.

After transmission of HIV, a high percentage of infected carriers will go on to develop a fatal illness. The virus replicates slowly but continuously, generally taking several years before it begins to attack and destroy the person's T-helper lymphocytes and macrophages. The destruction of these cells leads to deficiencies in multiple branches of the person's immune system. The incubation period for adults is between 6 months and 7 years. To date, the male homosexual population has the highest rate of infection in the United States. Other populations at high risk for infection include bisexual males, intravenous drug abusers, hemophiliacs who received contaminated blood products before 1985, and male or female sexual partners of persons in any of the previous groups. Pediatric AIDS cases differ from those in adults in that neonates acquire the infection from mothers who are infected. The onset of symptoms in such children generally occurs by the age of 2.

AIDS is not a single disease, but rather a collection of various diseases that characteristically develop in patients who are HIV positive. The HIV virus suppresses the immune system, making the patient susceptible to unusual **neoplasms** such as Kaposi's sarcoma, a wide variety of severe **opportunistic infections,** and neurologic disorders. The diagnosis of HIV infection in asymptomatic patients is made by testing for specific antibodies formed against the virus or by detecting the virus. Serologic tests in persons who have been infected with the HIV generally become positive within 2 months of exposure to the virus. It is very uncommon for an infected person to go more than 6 months without a detectable antibody response.

Since 1983, there have been several reported cases of transmission of the HIV to health care professionals; the majority of these followed a needlestick injury with contaminated blood. When compared with the total number of needlestick injuries reported by health care professionals, the number of HIV infections is low. It should be remembered that gloves provide protection against spillage and contamination only; they cannot protect the wearer from needlestick injury. However, gloves do protect phlebotomists when they have cuts, scratches, or other breaks in the skin.

Health care professionals caring for AIDS patients should be familiar with the types of infections seen in these patients so that appropriate protective measures can be employed when needed. The most common severe infectious complications of AIDS include infection with *Pneumocystis carinii* or *Toxoplasma gondii* organisms, *Mycobacterium avium* complex, infection with *Mycobacterium tuberculosis* organisms, cytomegalovirus, herpes simplex virus, HBV, and infection with *Salmonella* or *Cryptococcus* organisms.

PREVENTION

To date, no vaccine for AIDS has been developed, nor has a therapeutic cure been found. Preventive measures rely on the practice of infection control procedures as established by the CDC to prevent transmission of HIV infection to health care professionals. These guidelines, published in 1987, are known as the "Universal Blood and Body-Fluid Precautions,"[4] and are briefly outlined in Table 3–3. The CDC advises that health care organizations operate under the assumption that all patients are potentially infectious. (Previously, special precautions, such as the wearing of gloves while performing procedures, were used only

---

table **3-3**   **THE CDC's UNIVERSAL BLOOD AND BODY FLUID PRECAUTIONS: A BRIEF OUTLINE**

The Universal Blood and Body Fluid Precautions were designed to prevent parenteral, mucous membrane, and nonintact skin exposure to pathogens among health care practitioners. These guidelines are intended to supplement, not supplant, other recommendations for routine infection control practices. Briefly, the Universal Precautions are as follows:

Infectious fluids are defined as blood, blood products, semen and vaginal secretions, cerebrospinal fluid, synovial fluid, pleural fluid, peritoneal fluid, pericardial fluid, and amniotic fluid

Noninfectious fluids are defined as feces, nasal secretions, sputum, sweat, tears, urine, and vomit (unless blood is present)

Do not recap needles by hand; do not bend or manipulate used needles by hand

Exercise extra caution when using or cleaning any sharp instrument, such as needles, or other laboratory device

Dispose of all sharp items in puncture-resistant waste containers

Use protective barriers such as gloves, gowns, goggles, shields, and masks to prevent exposure to blood and other possibly infectious fluids and materials

Wash skin surfaces immediately and thoroughly after any exposure to an infectious fluid

---

From Centers for Disease Control: Recommendations for prevention of HIV transmission in health care settings. MMWR 36(suppl 2):15–185, 1987.

when the patient was considered to be a high-risk patient, such as an HIV-positive patient.) The CDC recommendations state that all health care workers should routinely use **barrier precautions** (i.e., gloves) whenever they are going to be in contact with blood, body fluids, mucous membranes, or the nonintact skin of a patient. A germicidal soap should be used to wash contaminated skin surfaces, and in the event of a spill, the environmental surfaces should be cleansed and decontaminated with a 1:10 dilution of household bleach.

Needlestick protection protocols have also been developed by the CDC to prevent the transmission of infection. Most accidental needlestick injuries occur while attempting to recap a used needle. The protocols therefore state that needles should not be recapped, but should be placed in puncture-proof containers that allow for disposal of the needle and syringe without having to recap or cut off the needle.

As the incidence of HIV-positive patients increases, so will the potential for transmission to health care professionals. Education and the use of protective measures are the keys to preventing exposure to AIDS and other infectious diseases.

Other Viral Infectious Diseases

INFLUENZA

Influenza virus A produces the most serious form of influenza, with symptoms of fever, chills, headache, myalgia, sore throat, and cough. The onset of symptoms is approximately 1 to 4 days after contact with infected respiratory secretions. Infected persons shed the virus for 24 hours before the onset of symptoms and for 3 to 4 days during the course of the disease. Death associated with this virus is usually the result of primary influenza pneumonia or a secondary bacterial pneumonia. The influenza viruses that are the cause of epidemics and nosocomial outbreaks change from season to season, and a new vaccine is manufactured each year.

Prevention. Vaccination, or a "flu shot," is recommended yearly for all health care personnel who have patient contact. Such a program will lower the risk of transmission of influenza from caregivers to patients and reduce the possibility of employee illness and absenteeism because of this virus.[2]

RUBELLA (GERMAN MEASLES)

Rubella, or German measles, generally produces only a mild illness in children and adults, but can cause congenital malformations if a woman is infected early in her pregnancy. Infection of the fetus can cause severe abnormalities, premature birth, or fetal death. Health care professionals are often young women, and the susceptibility rate in this age group is approximately 10% to 25%. In addition, the risk of contact between an infected professional and pregnant patients is ever present.

Transmission of rubella is from person to person by direct contact with infected respiratory secretions. There is a 2- to 3-week incubation period before symptoms are evident, but the virus begins to be shed from the throat of the patient during the first week after transmission.

Prevention. There is no specific antiviral treatment for rubella infection. Vaccination is recommended for all health care professionals who have no proof of previous vaccination or laboratory evidence of immunity.[2] Immunity is long lasting.

MUMPS AND MEASLES

Mumps is typically not a serious disease, but in a small percentage of cases, complications may be fatal. The most typical symptom is swelling of the parotid salivary glands. The virus is shed in the saliva during the 14- to 24-day incubation period and for about 9 days after the onset of symptoms.

Measles is a systemic infection that often causes a serious illness with pneumonia and secondary bacterial infections. Central nervous system involvement is present in many cases. Teens and young adults account for the majority of cases today. Illness begins with fever, cough, runny nose, and **conjunctivitis** and is characterized by a **maculopapular** rash and bright red spots with a central whitish dot (Koplik's spots) that develop inside the mouth. The measles virus multiplies in the respiratory tract, and infection is transmitted by respiratory secretions. Infected persons are most contagious during the incubation period and the early symptomatic period.

Prevention. Measles and mumps transmission in health care institutions can be disruptive and costly. To prevent such infections, the CDC recommends that all new personnel born in 1957 or later who have direct patient contact should be vaccinated. The measles-mumps-rubella vaccine (MMR) is the vaccine of choice. Persons born before 1957 are considered to be immune to both measles and mumps, because virtually everyone born before that time became infected naturally before the vaccine became available.[2]

POLIOVIRUS

The poliovirus, like other enteroviruses, is transmitted by the fecal-oral route or by respiratory secretions. Most persons infected with this virus are asymptomatic or experience only a mild illness. Poliovirus is shed in the feces for several weeks, and therefore, human feces are the source of virus in the environment. Respiratory shedding of the virus from the throat can last as long as 3 to 4 weeks. Polio is rare in countries such as the United States, and infection is generally limited to nonimmunized persons.

Prevention. There is no specific antiviral therapy for enteroviral infections such as polio. Effective poliovirus vaccines have been available since 1955, when the inactivated vaccine was released, and in 1962, the oral live **attenuated** vaccine was developed. Although live vaccine is less expensive and easier to administer, the virus multiplies, is shed in the feces, and represents a potential risk for transmission to others. Normally the poliovirus vaccine is not routinely recommended for persons older than 18 years. However, the CDC recommends that hospital personnel caring for patients who may be excreting wild polioviruses complete a primary series of poliovirus vaccine.[2]

SELECTED BACTERIAL INFECTIOUS DISEASES

Diseases Caused by Mycobacteria

Tuberculosis. Both normal individuals and immunocompromised patients (e.g., AIDS patients) may become infected with *M. tuberculosis,* the organism that causes tuberculosis. Tuberculosis is a chronic disease that most frequently produces lesions in the lungs, although disease may develop in other parts of the body. Infection normally occurs by the respiratory route. Patients with this disease are placed under respiratory precautions for the protection of the staff and visitors. Recently an antituberculosis drug–resistant strain of *Mycobacterium tuberculosis* has been reported. Successful treatment for patients infected with this strain may be problematic, requiring the use of multiple drugs.

Mycobacterium avium complex

AIDS patients frequently develop *M. avium* complex infection, which results in high numbers of organisms present in their blood and stool. Infection with these atypical mycobacteria causes AIDS patients to have bouts of diarrhea, as well as respiratory symptoms. Treatment of infection is extremely difficult, requiring multiple drug use because of the organism's high resistance to antituberculosis drugs.

Prevention. Depending on the species of mycobacteria involved in an infection, respiratory precautions (i.e., the use of a mask) as well as enteric precautions may be required. Antimycobacterial drugs are available and are effective in almost all cases except for the strains mentioned that have developed extreme drug resistance. Health care professionals, as part of their health protection program, should be tested before they begin working for previous exposure to mycobacteria. A purified protein derivative (PPD) of tubercle bacilli is used for this skin test. PPD testing should be done at yearly intervals during employment to check for any subsequent exposure to mycobacteria that would put the worker at risk for active infection.

Infection by *Salmonella, Shigella,* and *Campylobacter* Species

Salmonella, Shigella, and *Campylobacter* organisms characteristically cause diarrheal diseases. These infections are generally acquired by the oral-fecal route, being transmitted from person to person or in contaminated food or drink. Infected patients are placed on enteric precautions (i.e., the use of gloves and protective clothing), and infected employees are not permitted to have contact with patients or may be sent home until they have tested negative for these organisms. Typhoid fever is caused by one of the species of *Salmonella* and, as may be true for all of these bacteria, may persist in patients, who then become asymptomatic carriers. The feces of asymptomatic carriers are a more important source of contamination than the oral route in symptomatic patients placed on enteric precautions.

Prevention. Transmission of these organisms is most often by contact with the contaminated hands of health care personnel caring for an infected patient. Thorough hand washing before and after caring for patients is the most effective preventive measure. Effective antibiotic therapy is available for these infections, if necessary.

Staphylococcal Infection

The most pathogenic staphylococcus is *Staphylococcus aureus,* which characteristically causes localized abscess formation. *S. aureus* and *Staphylococcus epidermidis* are the most commonly isolated species in health care institutions. Both species are known to develop rapid antibacterial drug resistance. Infections with these strains are increasing in number, and hospitals are experiencing greater difficulty in treating patients with such infections. Contact spread of infection is an important consideration in hospitals, where large proportions of the staff and patients carry antibiotic-resistant *Staphylococcus* organisms in their noses or on their skin. The areas of the hospital where patients are at highest risk for severe staphylococcal infections are the newborn nursery, intensive care units, operating rooms, and chemotherapy units.

Prevention. Patients infected with staphylococci are placed under drainage and secretion precautions. Health care workers are thus alerted to the need for thorough hand-washing practices, as well as the use of gloves when in contact with areas of the patient's body. Staphylococci can be transmitted from contaminated linens and other objects in the environment, as well as directly from abscess secretions. Care should be used in placing equipment or transport devices on surfaces in the room that might contaminate them and thus spread the organism to the next room visited by the caregiver.

INFECTION CONTROL PRACTICES

Isolation Procedures

Isolation procedures were designed to prevent the transmission of infectious agents from patients to personnel or visitors and from personnel or visitors to patients. The precautions recommended for use in health care institutions depend both on the type of infection and on the patient's immunologic status. Infectious agents may be transmitted to patients via the airborne route or may be introduced by contaminated equipment or improper site preparation (as for venipuncture) or site selection. The risk of patient infection from venipuncture or capillary collection is low, although local site infections, as well as more serious infections such as bacteremia, have been associated with these procedures.

The CDC has established a category-specific isolation system that groups diseases for which similar isolation precautions are indicated.[5] Personnel and visitors are made aware of the need for special precautions by signs placed outside the patient's room. These signs describe the type of precaution required (e.g., "blood and body fluids") and the appropriate barrier precautions to be used by anyone entering the room (Fig. 3–1). Signs are also color coded for easy recognition. For their own protection, phlebotomists must become familiar with the various types of isolation precautions (Table 3–4). The specific isolation or precaution categories recommended for use in health care institutions by CDC are as follows:

Strict Isolation. This is designated for patients infected with highly contagious diseases, such as chickenpox, that are transmitted by respiratory secretions or infectious body substances. These patients are normally isolated in a private room. The use of a mask, gown, and gloves by personnel caring for these patients is required. Protective clothing should be put on before entering the room and should be carefully

PATIENT CARE

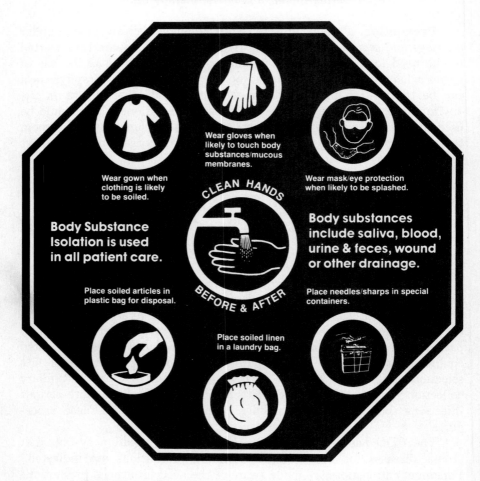

Wear gown when clothing is likely to be soiled.

Wear gloves when likely to touch body substances/mucous membranes.

Wear mask/eye protection when likely to be splashed.

CLEAN HANDS

Body Substance Isolation is used in all patient care.

Body substances include saliva, blood, urine & feces, wound or other drainage.

Place soiled articles in plastic bag for disposal.

BEFORE & AFTER

Place needles/sharps in special containers.

Place soiled linen in a laundry bag.

Body Substance Isolation

figure **3-1**   Sample isolation precaution sign. (Courtesy of Harborview Medical Center, Seattle, WA.)

removed and discarded in the appropriate container before leaving the area. Personnel should wash their hands thoroughly before and after leaving the room.

Respiratory Isolation. This is used to prevent transmission of infectious diseases, such as tuberculosis, that are spread through the air by droplets of respiratory secretions. Phlebotomists caring for such persons must wear a mask while they are in the room in addition to wearing gloves while performing the venipuncture procedure.

Enteric Precautions. These precautions indicate the need to protect personnel from microorganisms that are transmitted by direct or indirect contact with fecal material from the infected patient. Gloves and the protective clothing normally worn by phlebotomists while caring for patients provide adequate protection.

Drainage and Secretion Precautions. These protect personnel by preventing the transmission of infectious agents that are present in purulent material or drainage from an infected body site. Phlebotomists wearing protective clothing and gloves will be protected while caring for such patients and should not have to come in contact with areas where secretions are present.

Wound and Skin Precautions. For these precautions, the use of gloves is all that is required for phlebotomists, as they will not be drawing specimens from areas near wounds or infected skin surfaces. Nursing personnel and physicians are more at risk and are required to wear a gown and gloves.

Blood and Body Fluid Precautions. These precautions are perhaps the most important for phlebotomists. Although the Universal Precautions (see Table 3–3) technically eliminate the need for these special precautions, many hospitals have retained the use of this specific isolation category. Infections such as HIV, HBV, and HCV, which are transmitted by blood and other body fluids, are major occupational risks for health care providers. Indication of the need for precaution is designed to prevent contact with infective blood or body fluid. Gloves, as always, must be worn while performing venipuncture. A gown, mask, and goggles should be available if there is danger of splashing or spurting of blood.

Training in preventive measures will increase the confidence of professionals who care for infected patients. It is the responsibility of the health care institution to conduct in-service education programs in this area for personnel.

Patient Protection Precautions

A discussion of infection control is not complete unless consideration is given to those groups of patients who are at high risk of infection. Already compromised patients must be protected from infectious agents that might be transmitted by the phlebotomist. The most common high-risk patient areas or groups of patients are discussed below.

Nursery Units. Newborns do not have a fully developed immune system, and thus even healthy infants are at risk of infection. All persons intending to enter the nursery, including phlebotomists, must first wash table **3-4**   EXAMPLES OF DISEASES AND RECOMMENDED ISOLATION PRECAUTIONS

Strict isolation (yellow sign)
  Congenital rubella
  Diphtheria
  Herpes zoster
  Smallpox
  Varicella (chickenpox)
  Rabies

Enteric precautions (brown sign)
  Polio
  Cholera
  Rotavirus
  Minor wound infections
  Enteroviral infection
  Amebic dysentery
  Acute gastroenteritis

Wound and skin precautions (green sign)
  Staphylococcus aureus infections
  Group A Streptococcus infections
  Gas gangrene
  Scabies

Respiratory precautions (blue sign)
  Tuberculosis
  Measles
  Pertussis (whooping cough)
  Mumps
  Epiglottitis caused by Haemophilus infection
  Rubella
  Meningitis caused by meningococcus or Haemophilus infection

Drainage and secretion precautions (green sign)
  Leprosy
  Common cold
  Mucocutaneous candidiasis
  Herpes simplex
  Scarlet fever
  Toxic shock syndrome
  Infectious mononucleosis
  Chancroid

Blood and body fluid precautions (pink sign)
  Hepatitis infections
  HIV infections
  Syphilis—primary and secondary
  Lyme disease
  Rocky mountain spotted fever

their hands thoroughly and put on a gown, mask, and gloves. Only the equipment needed to perform the procedure should be taken into the nursery.

The protocol for gowning is as follows: A clean gown is put on with the opening in the back, and then both the neck strings and those at the waist are tied (Table 3–5). If a mask is required, it should be tied high on the head and also behind the head to prevent it from slipping. Gloves are the last barrier protection to be put on and should be pulled on so that the ends fit over the sleeves of the gown. (Table 3–6). After the patient procedure has been completed, the phlebotomist should leave the unit, remove all protective clothing, and dispose of it in the receptacle provided. Before leaving, the hands should be washed thoroughly once again.

Immunocompromised Patients. Protective or reverse isolation is designed to protect severely immunocompromised patients, who are highly susceptible to infectious diseases that may be transmitted to them

---

table **3-5**   GOWNING TECHNIQUE

---

1. Wash hands thoroughly
2. Put the gown on with the opening in the back; if a sterile gown is needed, only the inside of the gown should be touched as it is being put on.
3. Tie the strings in the back, at the neck and the waist.
4. The sleeves should be pulled down to the wrists.
5. Before removing the gown, wash hands thoroughly again.
6. To remove, untie the neck and then the waist of the gown.
7. The gown should be removed and folded with the contaminated side facing inward.
8. Place the folded gown in the specified receptacle.
9. Wash hands once more.

---

by other persons. Immunocompromised patients include bone marrow transplant patients, burn victims, leukemia patients, chemotherapy recipients, and organ transplant patients. Persons entering these areas or rooms should be gowned, gloved, and masked and should take with them only that equipment needed to perform the procedure. In some instances only presterilized materials may be taken into these rooms.

Intensive Care Units. These units care for the most seriously ill patients. Some patients may have an infectious disease and therefore are normally kept in a separate section of the unit, whereas other patients are recovering from surgical procedures and are being given drugs that reduce their ability to combat infection. Phlebotomists as well as other

---

table **3-6**   MASK AND GLOVE TECHNIQUES

Mask technique
1. Remove a mask from the box.
2. Place the mask over the nose and mouth.
3. First tie the upper tie high on the head to keep the mask in place; then tie the lower tie.
4. The mask should be removed after removing the gown and washing the hands again thoroughly.
5. Touch only the strings when removing the mask.
6. Discard in the designated receptacle.

Glove technique
1. Gloves are put on last and removed first.
2. Gloves need not be sterile.
3. Pull the ends of the gloves over the sleeves of the gown if a gown is required.
4. Jewelry, such as rings, that might puncture a glove should be removed.
5. Gloves should be discarded after each patient.
6. Hands should be washed after the gloves are removed.
7. Gloves are worn for all contact with blood and other body fluids.

---

health care providers should determine the need for barrier precautions other than gloves, which should always be worn, before they approach patients.

Blood Culture Collection and Bacteremia

Phlebotomists play a key role in the prompt and accurate isolation of the etiologic agents in cases of **bacteremia.** Bacteremia is one of the most critical aspects of an infectious disease. The identification of the agents of bacteremia is a primary function of the clinical microbiology laboratory. The ability of the laboratory to perform this task well is directly influenced by the quality of specimens submitted. The phlebotomists who collect the blood cultures determine the quality of these critical specimens. Numerous cases of bacteremia occur each year, and the associated mortality rate may be as high as 50%. *S. aureus* and *Escherichia coli* are the two microorganisms most commonly recovered from cultures of blood. The number of bacteria circulating in the patient's blood is usually low, and the blood culture systems used are designed to amplify the number of bacteria for easier detection. False-positive results caused by contamination result in prolonged patient hospitalizations, unnecessary and expensive antibiotic treatment, and additional costs for laboratory testing. There is a lower contamination rate and greater consistency in technique in those institutions where trained phlebotomists collect the blood cultures.

Careful preparation of the patient's arm is the most critical step. The skin is normally colonized by microorganisms such as staphylococci, streptococci, corynebacteria, and bacilli. The procedure for preparation of the site (see Chapter 6) is designed to destroy the organisms present on the skin so that they are not introduced into the culture system, amplified, and reported as a positive finding. The alcohol used kills bacteria and cleans the dirt and skin debris from the pores. Povidone-iodine (Betadine) or plain iodine is applied next, and also acts to kill most of the normal skin flora. Once the site has been prepared, the phlebotomist must ensure that the site is not touched unless sterile gloves are worn.

Of all the factors that influence the successful recovery of bacteria from the blood, the most important is the volume of blood collected for each culture. Phlebotomists must be familiar with the culture system used at their institution and the recommended volume of blood to be collected. Phlebotomists play an important role in patient care, and collection of blood specimens for cultures is perhaps their most important service to their patients.

Review
Questions

1. _____ is the most effective preventive measure to eliminate the transmission of disease in health care institutions.
2. The most frequently reported occupation-associated infection for persons who handle blood is _____.
3. Postexposure prophylaxis for a nonimmune health care professional exposed to HBV includes administration of the hepatitis B vaccine and hepatitis B _____.
4. The human immunodeficiency virus is the etiologic agent of the disease _____.
5. Most accidental needlestick injuries occur while attempting to _____ a used needle.

References

1. Centers for Disease Control: Public Health Service inter-agency guidelines for screening donors of blood, plasma, organs, tissues, and semen for evidence of hepatitis B and hepatitis C. MMWR 40(RR-4):1–13, 1991.
2. Centers for Disease Control: Update on adult immunization—recommendations of the Immunization Practices Advisory Committee (ACIP). MMWR 40(RR-12):5–7, 1991.
3. Centers for Disease Control: Hepatitis B virus: A comprehensive strategy for eliminating transmission in the United States through universal childhood vaccination. MMWR 40(RR-13):14, 1991.
4. Centers for Disease Control: Recommendations for prevention of HIV transmission in health care settings. MMWR 36(suppl 2):15–185, 1987.
5. Berg R: The APIC Curriculum for Infection Control Practice. Vol III. Dubuque, Iowa, Kendall/Hunt, 1988, pp 1162–1163.

Equipment

John C. Flynn, Jr.

Phlebotomists often hear that a blood test result can only be as good as the collected specimen. This includes, in addition to proper collection technique, proper evacuated tube selection and proper needle selection. If a hematology specimen is collected in a chemistry tube, then the sample is probably going to be worthless for hematologic analysis. Therefore, it is very important that the proper tube, along with the proper additive, is used in every blood collection.

This chapter will discuss the various tubes, their **anticoagulants,** and the other common equipment associated with phlebotomy and microcollection procedures.

TUBES AND ANTICOAGULANTS

Lavender-Stoppered Tubes

In the hematology laboratory, the majority of specimens are collected in *lavender-stoppered* (or purple-stoppered) tubes. The primary additive

59

in these tubes is the anticoagulant ethylenediaminetetra-acetate **(EDTA).** EDTA prevents blood from clotting by chelating or binding calcium. Calcium is needed for clot formation, and by binding calcium, coagulation can be prevented.

Lavender-stoppered tubes are used for general hematologic studies such as the complete blood cell **(CBC)** count, white blood cell **(WBC) differential,** and platelet count and function tests. Ideally, the blood smear for the WBC differential should be made from a drop of blood collected via a finger stick. However, this is usually not practical, and the EDTA tube is used. The smear should be made within ½ hour of the collection, because EDTA may cause some distortion of WBC morphology.

Blue-Stoppered Tubes

Another common tube used for the hematology laboratory (or, more precisely, the coagulation laboratory) is the *blue-stoppered* tube. Sodium citrate is used as the primary ingredient in these tubes to prevent coagulation. Sodium citrate, like EDTA, binds calcium and thus prevents coagulation. Blue-stoppered tubes are used for coagulation studies such as **prothrombin time** (PT) and **activated partial thromboplastin time** (PTT). Blood from these tubes cannot be used for CBC counts or differentials because of the effects of citrate on the cellular components.

Green-Stoppered Tubes

Green-stoppered tubes contain the anticoagulant sodium heparin or lithium heparin. Heparin is a natural anticoagulant and stops the coagulation process by inactivating thrombin and thromboplastin. Blood collected in these tubes is assayed when plasma or whole blood is needed — as, for example, in tests for ammonia. Green-stoppered tubes are also the tube of choice when doing human leukocyte antigen (HLA) typing or chromosome analysis.

Gray-Stoppered Tubes

To inhibit glycolytic action, sodium fluoride or sodium fluoride and thymol may be used. One of these ingredients is often combined with potassium oxalate, which inhibits the clotting process by binding calcium. These ingredients are found in *gray-stoppered* evacuation tubes. Blood collected in these tubes is generally used for glucose analysis or when whole blood is needed.

Yellow-Stoppered Tubes

Yellow-stoppered tubes often contain acid-citrate-dextrose (ACD). In addition to inhibiting the coagulation process, ACD maintains red blood cell viability. Yellow-stoppered tubes may also contain sodium polyanetholesulfonate (SPS). Tubes with SPS are often the tube of choice for blood culture collections.

Red-Stoppered Tubes and "Tiger Tops"

Tubes with *red-stoppers* are used very frequently. These tubes have no additive and are used when serum is required for testing, such as in blood banking procedures and many serology procedures. A special type of red-stoppered tube contains a serum-cell separator. These tubes have stoppers that are red and green, and they are often referred to as "tiger tops" or "speckled reds." The separator works by settling between the clot and the serum during centrifugation, thereby making it easier for the laboratory worker to access the serum. The tubes are used frequently in chemistry for a wide variety of tests. Becton-Dickinson (Rutherford, NJ) has marketed a tube with a serum-cell gel separator and a dry clot enhancer coated on the inside of the tube. Although the stopper is red, it has a gold plastic cap over it; otherwise it is used like the more traditional "tiger top" tube. This tube is referred to as a Hemoguard and will be discussed further at the end of this section.

Tubes With Other Colored Stoppers

Occasionally, tubes with other colored stoppers, such as black and dark blue, may be used. These may come with a variety of additives, so the phlebotomist should be aware of the additive these tubes contain before using them to collect a blood specimen. See the color plate for a listing of common stopper colors, anticoagulants, mode of action, and tests ordered.

Tube Size

Tubes may come in a variety of sizes, from 15 ml down to capillary sizes for microcapillary collections. The actual volume of blood collected

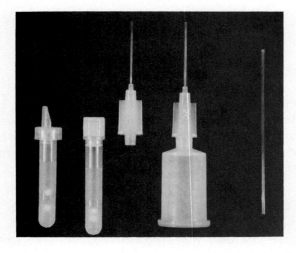

figure **4−1**

Microcollection tubes.

is dependent on the vacuum. For many tests that use a tube with an anticoagulant, a minimum amount of blood must be drawn into the tube. Otherwise the blood-to-anticoagulant ratio will not be ideal and this could adversely affect the test. The phlebotomist should check the manufacturer's specifications regarding the minimal acceptable amount of blood that can be drawn into an anticoagulated tube.

Most tubes used for adults will range from 3 to 10 ml. Pediatric evacuated tubes generally range from 2 to 4 ml. Blood-holding devices for microcapillary collection hold less than 1 ml of blood. Figure 4−1 shows some examples of blood-collecting tubes for microcapillary collection.

Splashguards

In an effort to reduce the aerosol mist that may be generated when a stopper is removed from a tube, a stopper has been manufactured that has a plastic splashguard placed over the rubber stopper. A tube with this type of stopper is known as a Hemoguard (Fig. 4−2). Hemoguard tubes are available as replacements for all of the commonly used traditional tubes. The splashguard decreases the aerosol mist, which may be infectious. Also, some tubes are designed so that certain instruments can access the specimen directly, thus entirely eliminating the need to remove the stopper.

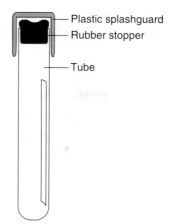

Plastic splashguard
Rubber stopper
Tube

figure **4–2**

Cross section of a collection tube with a splashguard, which is used to reduce the potentially infectious aerosol mist that may be generated when the stopper is removed from the tube.

NEEDLES

A very important part of the blood collection system is the needle. Needles are hollow stainless steel shafts with a beveled end. Each needle is sterilized and individually packaged. In many countries needles are reused after cleaning and sterilization, but in the United States all needles are used once and then disposed of properly.

Needle Size

Needles come in a variety of sizes, which is referred to as the *needle gauge*. The gauge is a measurement of the diameter of the needle: the larger the gauge number, the smaller the diameter of the needle. For routine phlebotomy, most needles are 21 or 22 gauge; however, during blood donation, an 18-gauge needle is common. If a patient has small or fragile veins, the phlebotomist will want to use a small gauge (for example, a 22-gauge needle).

Needles are generally 1 or 1½ inches in length. The needle selected will depend on the individual patient and on the depth of the vein from which blood is to be collected.

Multiple-Draw Needles

Another variable in needle choice is whether the needle will be used for a single draw or multiple draw. In other words, will one or more than

Retractable sheath during blood collection

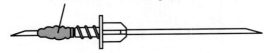

Retractable sheath when no tube is engaged

Bevel end

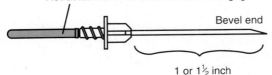

1 or 1½ inch

figure **4–3**

Multidraw needle demonstrating the retractable sheath.

one tube of blood be collected? The multiple-draw needle has a retractable sheath over the part of the needle that extends into the evacuated tube. This sheath prevents blood from leaking out while the phlebotomist is changing tubes. Figure 4–3 demonstrates how a multiple-draw needle works.

Butterfly Needles

Although generally used as part of an intravenous set to administer fluids or medicine to patients, the butterfly needle (Fig. 4–4) is sometimes used to collect blood from difficult patients. Once the butterfly

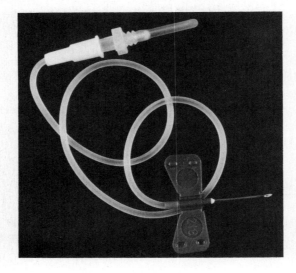

figure **4–4**

Butterfly needle.

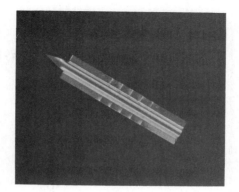

figure **4-5**

Microlance.

needle is in place, a syringe or evacuated tube, with a tube holder, is used to withdraw blood from the vein.

Blood Lancets

For difficult patients, including situations that normally call for microcapillary techniques, a blood lancet may be used. This is a small, sterile, disposable instrument used for skin puncture (Fig. 4–5). Lancets are available with a variety of point lengths to help control the depth of puncture, which is especially important in children and infants. A variety of semiautomated lancet devices are commercially available, but the manual lancet is the most commonly used device for microcapillary puncture.

Needle Disposal Equipment

Needle disposal equipment has evolved over time from manually recapping and then unscrewing needles, to cutting off the needle, and finally, to unscrewing the needle directly into a puncture-proof container. The purpose is to avoid any accidental needle punctures, and therefore, the less the phlebotomist has to directly manipulate the needle, the less possibility there is of needle puncture. The puncture-proof containers come in a variety of sizes; some are small enough to fit conveniently on the phlebotomist's tray. Figure 4–6 demonstrates how the needle is unscrewed into a disposal container. Other needle safety and disposal devices are commercially available to prevent accidental needle punctures, but the puncture-proof containers are the most popular devices currently in use.

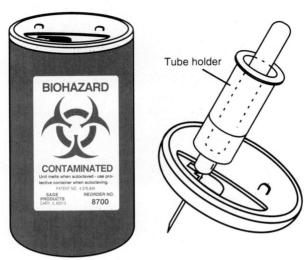

figure **4-6** Needle disposal container. The inset shows the hub of the needle seated into the lid. The needle is unscrewed and allowed to drop into the receptacle, which can be permanently closed when filled.

TUBE HOLDERS

The tube holder, or, as it is sometimes called, the barrel, allows the phlebotomist to safely and securely manipulate the evacuated tubes and draw blood from a patient. Holders come in a variety of sizes to accomodate the variety of evacuated tubes. Figure 4-7 shows a fully assembled needle, tube, and tube holder.

TOURNIQUETS

The purpose of the tourniquet is to increase resistance in the venous blood flow. When this happens, the veins become distended and can be more easily **palpated** or located. However, the tourniquet should not remain on the patient too long (1 to 2 minutes maximum), because this could adversely affect the test results as well as be uncomfortable for the patient. There are a variety of tourniquets available, including blood pressure cuffs, rubber tubing, and rubber straps.

Although a blood pressure cuff is an ideal tourniquet because the pressure can be accurately regulated, it is not practical to use for routine venipunctures. However, when confronted with a difficult "stick," a blood pressure cuff is very helpful. The more commonly used tourniquet is the rubber strap, which is tied in a slip loop (see Chapter 5) above the

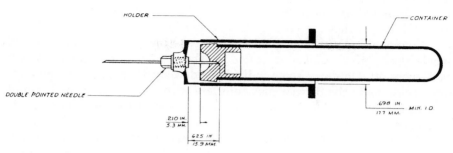

POSITION 1
PREPARATION FOR VENIPUNCTURE

HOLDER

CONTAINER

DOUBLE POINTED NEEDLE

.698 IN
17.7 MM. MIN. I.D.

210 IN.
5.3 MM.

.625 IN
15.9 MM.

NOTES:

1 NEEDLE TO LOCK IN PLACE WITH MATING HOLDER

2 STOPPER DIMENSIONS TO ALLOW FOR TWO
POSITIONS AS SHOWN.

POSITION 2
COLLECTION OF SPECIMEN

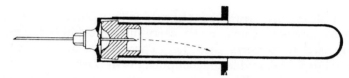

figure **4–7**   Fully assembled venipuncture set. (Reproduced with permission from H1-A3, "Evacuated Tubes for Blood Specimen Collection — Third Edition; Approved Standard," National Committee for Chemical Laboratory Standards, 711 E. Lancaster Avenue, Villanova, PA 19085.)

venipuncture site. Some rubber straps are equipped with Velcro, thereby eliminating the need for the slip loop. Penrose tubing is occasionally used, but the rubber strap is generally the tourniquet of choice.

GLOVES

With the implementation of the Occupational Safety and Health Administration (OSHA) regulations for blood-borne pathogens and the advent of Universal Precautions, gloves have become mandatory in blood collection. They provide a protective barrier between the phlebotomist and any infectious agents that could enter the body through a cut or abrasion. Remember, just because cuts or abrasions cannot be seen does not mean they are not present. *There is no excuse for not using gloves.*

Gloves are made from a variety of materials, but the most commonly used materials are vinyl, latex, and nitrile. Vinyl gloves are probably the least desirable, because they do not fit snugly and do not conform to the shape of the individual's hand. Latex gloves are the most commonly used, because they fit nicely and conform to the individual's hand. Many phlebotomists prefer the nitrile gloves. These have a fit similar to that of latex gloves but are more tear resistant and feel more comfortable on the hand. However, they are slightly more expensive.

Commonly, gloves are available with talcum powder lightly dusted inside them, which makes it easier for the wearer to put them on and take them off. However, some individuals develop allergies to the powder, and occasionally the powder may interfere with some tests or be harmful to sensitive equipment. For these situations, powder-free gloves are available from a variety of vendors.

Finally, gloves are available in dispenser boxes or are individually wrapped and sterilized, which is more costly. Generally, dispenser boxes are most commonly encountered in phlebotomy units.

PHLEBOTOMY TRAYS

Phlebotomy trays are commercially available carriers that enable phlebotomists to conveniently carry all the equipment and supplies they may need to perform their job. These trays are generally carried, but some hospitals provide phlebotomists with push carts on which they may place their trays. The trays must allow the phlebotomist to carry an adequate supply of all of the previously mentioned equipment. See Figure 4–8 for a picture of a fully stocked phlebotomy tray.

OTHER COMMON SUPPLIES

Other common supplies that the phlebotomist will need are alcohol pads, gauze, surgical tape, pens, ammonia salts, and adhesive bandages. Table 4–1 lists the common equipment that a phlebotomist may need.

table **4–1**   COMMON EQUIPMENT A PHLEBOTOMIST SHOULD CARRY

Needles (various sizes and microcapillary)
Evacuated tubes (various sizes and colors)
Microcapillary collection equipment
Tube holders
Tourniquets
Alcohol swabs
Gauze
Adhesive bandages or tape
Gloves
Sharps containers
Marking pens
Clay sealer

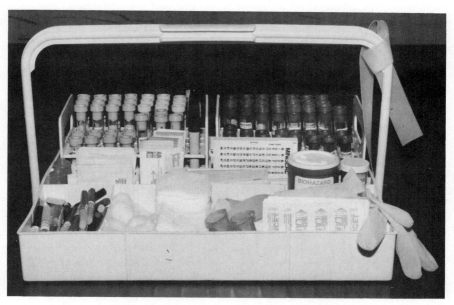

figure **4–8**   Fully stocked phlebotomy tray.

chapter **Four**	# Review Questions

1. The anticoagulant in a lavender top tube is _____.
2. A small, sterile, disposable instrument used for skin puncture is the _____.
3. _____ are disposed of in puncture-proof containers.
4. The rubber strap is a type of _____.
5. In an effort to reduce aerosol mist, a _____ is placed over the rubber stopper by some manufacturers.

Proper Procedures for Venipuncture

John C. Flynn, Jr.

chapter Outline

Patient Greeting and Identification	Physiologic and Biologic Considerations
Routine Venipuncture	
Microcapillary Blood Collection	

The previous chapter discussed the equipment and anticoagulants used in common blood collection techniques. In this chapter, the actual techniques practiced in evacuated tube and microcapillary collections, beginning with greeting and identifying the patient and continuing through to labeling and transporting the specimen, will be discussed and illustrated. (Syringe collection technique will be discussed in a subsequent chapter.)

PATIENT GREETING AND IDENTIFICATION

The manner in which a phlebotomist greets a patient can often set the tone for the remainder of the phlebotomy procedure. A later chapter is devoted to interpersonal communication and professionalism, but it must be emphasized here that phlebotomists must always conduct themselves in a professional manner. Therefore, when greeting a patient, be courteous and respectful. Treat them the way you would like to be treated. Additionally, if the patient's door is shut when you get to the room, knock and listen for a response before you enter. Of course, this may not always be feasible, depending on the patient and the surrounding circumstances.

After greeting the patient, one of the most important steps in venipuncture—possibly the most important—is proper patient identification. Identification can be both visual and verbal. When you enter a patient's room, you will generally have certain information such as the patient's name, identification number, and age or date of birth. Compare the information you have with the patient's physical appearance and the identification bracelet. For example, if your requisition lists the patient's name as Sarah Jones and you encounter a male patient, there is a problem. Do not use the information on the chart attached to the bed or on the name plate on or above the bed. Patients may be transferred, and name plates may not be accurate. The only dependable information is on the patient's wristband. Also, it is best to ask patients to state their name rather than having them respond to a question. For example, it is best to say, "Please tell me your full name," rather than, "Are you Mrs. Jones?" If the patient is incoherent or has difficulty hearing, they may answer "yes," no matter what they are asked, in an effort to be cooperative.

ROUTINE VENIPUNCTURE

This section will discuss the proper procedure for performing routine venipuncture. Remember, as in the illustrations, *gloves must be worn at all times.*

POSITIONING (Fig. 5–1).   Position the patient's arm in such a way that it is comfortable for both you and the patient and you have clear access to the antecubital area. The arm should be supported by a firm surface such as an armrest on a chair or on the bed if the patient is lying down.

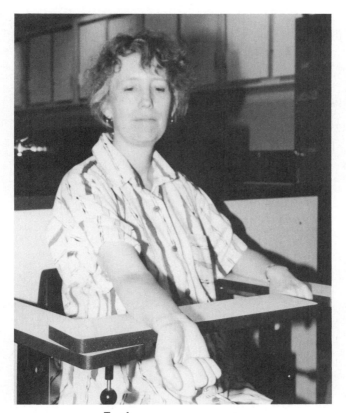

figure **5-1** A properly supported arm.

2 **APPLYING THE TOURNIQUET (**Fig. 5-2).   Once the arm is positioned, place the tourniquet firmly about the upper arm. The tourniquet needs to be tight enough to increase blood pressure in the veins but not so tight that it cuts off the circulation. Figure 5-2 shows how the tourniquet should be tied. After some practice, you will learn how to adjust the tourniquet for proper snugness. The tourniquet should never remain on the patient's arm for more than 1 to 2 minutes.

Proper method for tying a tourniquet

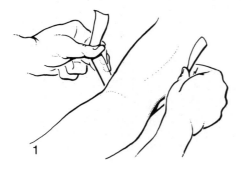

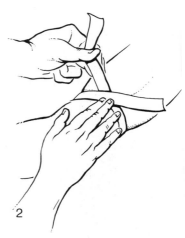

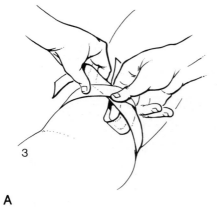

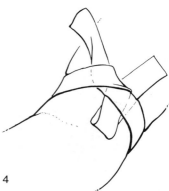

A

Tourniquet in place

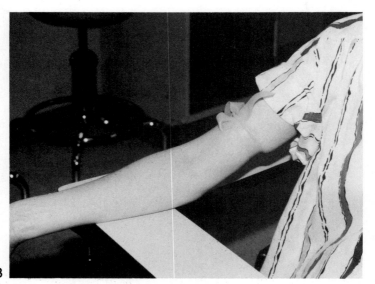

B

figure **5-2**   *A, B,* Tourniquet application.

3

CHOOSING THE SITE (Fig. 5–3).   Try to locate the median cubital vein (generally the largest and best anchored vein, near the center of the antecubital area). Other veins that may be acceptable are the cephalic and the basilic veins (see Figure

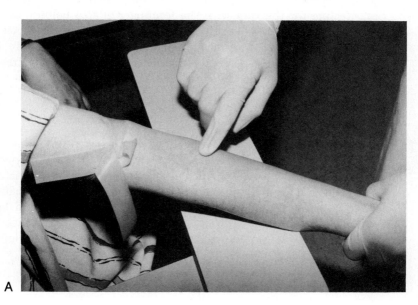

A

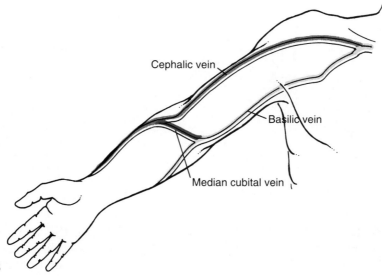

Cephalic vein

Basilic vein

Median cubital vein

B

figure **5–3**   *A, B,* Locating a vein.

5–3*B*). Veins in the back of the hand may also be acceptable, but in these cases it is wise to use pediatric needles and evacuated tubes. To enhance visualization of the veins, position the arm at a downward angle, using the force of gravity as an aid. Also, rubbing the forearm toward the antecubital area, instructing the patient to make a fist, may enhance vein visualization. Palpating and feeling for the vein with the forefinger is also helpful; do not forget that you can look on both arms before you make a decision and that there will be times when you cannot see the vein but can feel it. The prospective venipuncture site should be free of skin abrasions, lesions, and scar tissue.

4 **ASSEMBLING THE EQUIPMENT** (Fig. 5–4). Assemble the needle, the barrel, and the first tube you wish to use. The needle should not be uncovered until ready to perform venipuncture. Place any additional tubes to be used in a convenient location, keeping some spares handy. The gauze, alcohol pads, and bandages should be ready. (*Note:* Some phlebotomists may elect to do this step before applying the tourniquet; this is acceptable.)

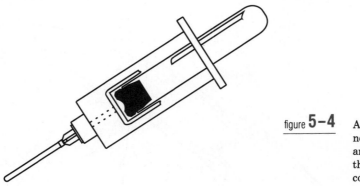

figure **5–4** An assembled needle, holder, and tube; note that needle is uncovered.

5 **CLEANSING THE SITE** (Fig. 5–5). Cleanse the venipuncture site with 70% isopropyl alcohol by making outward concentric circles. *This must be allowed to dry,* either by air drying or by using clean gauze. *Once the site is cleansed, it must not be touched;* if touched, it must be recleansed.

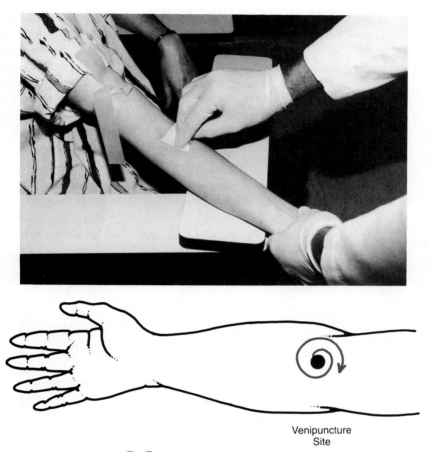

Venipuncture
Site

figure **5-5**   Cleansing the venipuncture site.

6 **PERFORMING THE VENIPUNCTURE** (Fig. 5-6).   With the bevel up, quickly and smoothly insert the needle into the vein and engage the evacuated tube.

(Special note: There is no right way or wrong way to hold the needle and adapter for venipuncture. Phlebotomy instructors may advocate one way over another because of familiarity and experience. The phlebotomy student must discover which way is most comfortable and which yields the best results.)

Be sure to stretch the skin surrounding the venipuncture before inserting the needle; this will aid in anchoring the vein and will make needle insertion less painful. Never tell patients that they will not feel the needle puncture or that it will not hurt. Be honest with the patient. If no blood is immediately forthcoming, slight manipulation of the needle may be helpful; you may have gone in too deep, not deep enough, or to one side of the vein. Avoid "probing," and do not attempt a venipuncture more than two times on a given patient. (See Chapter 7 for a more thorough discussion on what to do if you do not obtain blood.)

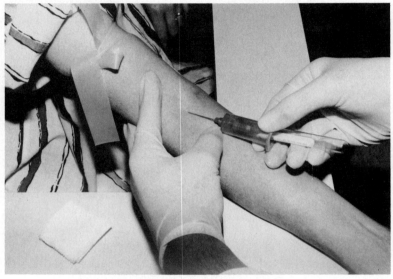

figure **5-6** Venipuncture.

7 **RELEASING THE TOURNIQUET** (Fig. 5-7). Once good blood flow is established and before the final tube is filled, release the tourniquet. If the tourniquet was applied properly, you should be able to release it with a simple tug.

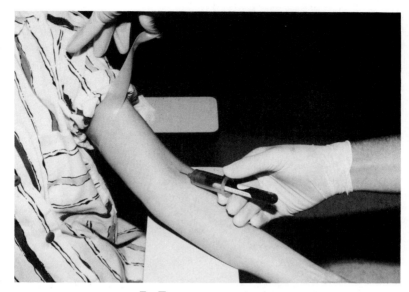

figure **5−7**   Releasing the tourniquet.

8 **REMOVING THE NEEDLE** (Fig. 5–8).   Once the last tube of blood is filled and you have removed it from the needle and tube holder, you may remove the needle. Do this in a single smooth, swift motion, and quickly apply clean gauze over the puncture site. If the patient is able, instruct him or her to apply pressure

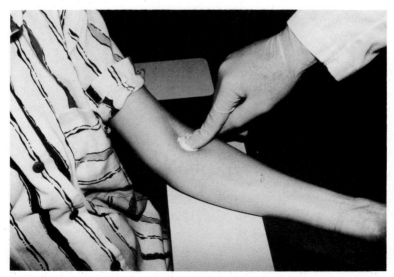

figure **5−8**   Applying pressure after needle removal.

and to keep the arm straight. If the patient is unable to do this, it is the phlebotomist's responsibility to apply pressure until the bleeding has stopped. Outpatients may use a bandage to cover the venipuncture site, but hospitals may have different policies about using bandages on inpatients. Be sure you are familiar with the policies at your institution.

9   **NEEDLE DISPOSAL** (Fig. 5–9).   Properly dispose of your needle. *Do not lay it down, and do not recap it.*

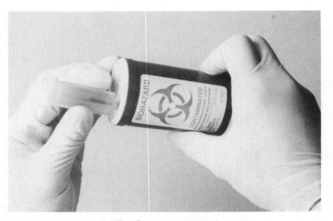

figure **5–9**   Needle disposal.

10   **SPECIMEN LABELING AND TRANSPORTATION** (Fig. 5–10). Immediately label the specimen. If any specimens require mixing (e.g., in blue- or purple-stoppered tubes), do so by gently inverting the tubes several times. Regarding labeling, remember that the patient's wristband is the primary source of information. In some hospitals, certain specimens (e.g., those for the blood bank) must be hand labeled and initialed by the phlebotomist. Therefore, be familiar with any special labeling requirements at your

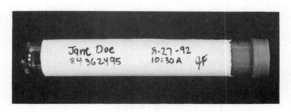

figure **5–10**

Properly labeled specimen.

institution. Also, as a responsible phlebotomist, you must be aware of any special transportation requirements. Does the specimen need to be transported on ice (e.g., for an ammonia test)? Does the specimen need to be maintained at 37°C (e.g., for a cold agglutinin test)? Is the specimen a STAT (i.e., needing immediate analysis)? Be familiar with any special transportation requirements before collecting the blood specimen.

11 **HAND WASHING** (Fig. 5–11).   Before moving on to the next patient, remove and properly discard your gloves, and then thoroughly wash your hands.

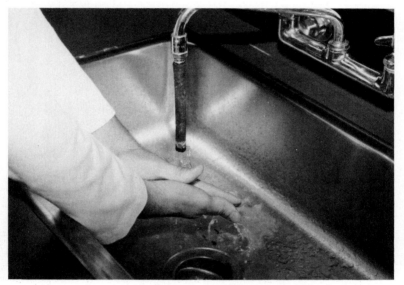

figure **5–11**   Hand washing.

Occasionally, venipuncture must be performed on a young child or toddler. The equipment and procedure are basically the same as for an adult patient, but the child may need some restraint. See Chapter 7 for further discussion and illustration of performing phlebotomy on a child.

MICROCAPILLARY BLOOD COLLECTION

Microcapillary blood collections are used primarily when the patient has no adequate veins for venipuncture, either because of age (very young or very old) or for some other reason, such as burns or dermatitis.

Obviously the amount of blood collected will be much smaller than that collected via venipuncture, which in turn means the physician must be very sure of the tests he or she wishes to be performed.

The technique for microcapillary collection is not drastically different from the venipuncture technique described earlier. Gloves are used at all times. The site of the skin puncture is usually the finger but may also be the earlobe or the heel in the case of an infant (discussed further in Chapter 6). No tourniquet is applied, but instead the site is held firmly by the phlebotomist. Figure 5–12A shows how to hold a finger to perform

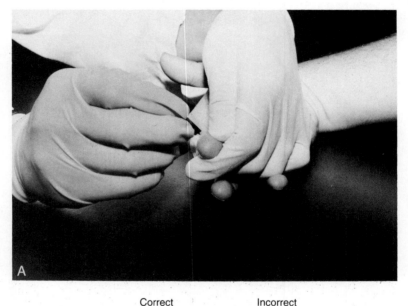

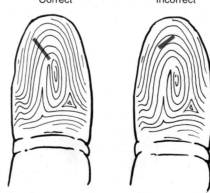

Correct   Incorrect

figure **5-12**   *A*, An accepted way to hold a finger for skin puncture. *B*, The skin puncture in a finger stick should be perpendicular to the lines of the fingerprint.

a skin puncture. Site preparation is identical, but a microlance is used instead of a needle and tube (see Fig. 4–5). When doing a finger stick, make the puncture off the center of the finger and perpendicular to the lines of the fingerprint (Fig. 5–12*B*). It is important to remember to wipe away the first drop of blood, because the blood in this drop will be diluted with tissue fluid, which could alter the laboratory results. Some variation of a microcollection tube is used to collect the blood (see Fig. 4–1). At the completion of the blood collection, either the phlebotomist or the patient must maintain pressure on the puncture site until bleeding has stopped. All used material is properly disposed of—the lancet in the puncture-proof container and the used gauze and gloves in a biohazard receptacle. As in venipuncture, hands must be washed before going to the next patient.

General Considerations

The following general considerations apply to blood collection either by venipuncture or by skin puncture.

1. Always act professionally and be considerate of the patient.
2. Never quarrel with a patient.
3. Use expendable equipment, such as needles, lancets, and gauze, only once.
4. Avoid venipuncture more than two times on a given patient.
5. Always wear gloves.
6. Never recap needles, but dispose of them properly.

PHYSIOLOGIC AND BIOLOGIC CONSIDERATIONS

Occasionally, laboratory testing of a blood sample will result in a spurious result or be considered a "mistake" by a physician in the laboratory or nurse on the floor. Actually what has occurred is a variation from the **basal state** of the patient, which has influenced the **analyte**. Any number of things can interfere with the basal state of a patient (e.g., diet, exercise, stress, trauma, or change in posture). The time of day can also interfere with the baseline results one would expect to obtain on testing.

Diet is probably the most obvious factor that may affect testing. This is especially true when analyses for glucose or triglycerides are performed. The importance of collecting fasting or timed specimens is discussed more fully in Chapter 6, but it is important to note the time a specimen is collected and whether it is a fasting specimen.

The level of certain enzymes, such as creatine phosphokinase (CPK), in the blood may help diagnose heart damage. However, this same enzyme is also found in all other muscle tissue. If the patient has engaged in moderate to strenuous *exercise* in the 24 hours preceding the collection of the blood specimen, an elevated level of the enzyme, not related to a heart condition, may be found. (It should be noted that if an elevated CPK level is encountered, a more specific test should be performed.) Exercise may also affect the levels of other enzymes as well as various hemostatic factors. For the phlebotomist, it may be wise to note whether a patient has engaged in exercise in the 24 hours preceding blood collection.

Stress caused by the anticipation of having a blood specimen collected may alter the levels of certain constituents in the blood. For example, white blood cells may increase if the patient is overanxious about the phlebotomy. Therefore, it is best — and easier — to collect the specimen when the patient is calm.

The *trauma* associated with an accident will adversely affect the results of some tests. If the muscles are injured in a traumatic accident, CPK will be released into the blood system and may initially give a false indication of heart trouble.

A change in posture may not only change blood pressure, it may also significantly alter the results obtained when testing for certain analytes such as proteins, lipids, iron, and enzymes. This is especially true when a patient has been in one position for a period of time and blood is collected shortly after he or she changes position.

Finally, the *time of day* that a specimen is collected will affect the results of testing. Serum cortisol, used to monitor adrenal function, is notably affected by circadian rhythm, again illustrating the importance of noting the time that a blood specimen is collected.

table **5-1**	HEMOGLOBIN VALUES ACCORDING TO AGE AND GENDER
	Normal Hemoglobin Value (gm/dl)
Newborn	17–23
2-month-old child	9–14
Adult male	14–18
Adult female	12–16

In addition to the physiologic variations mentioned earlier, certain biologic conditions may affect testing results. These include factors such as age, sex, race, and pregnancy. If appropriate, laboratories generally have different sets of normal values depending on what test is being performed. Table 5–1 shows how normal values for hemoglobin may vary. Often the age, sex, and race are noted on requisition slips or computer-generated labels. If not, it will be very informative to the laboratory if the phlebotomist provides this information, in addition to noting whether the patient is pregnant.

The above paragraphs mention only a few of the many blood constituents that may be affected by a variety of physiologic and biologic conditions. For phlebotomists, any information that can be provided to the laboratory to help explain spurious results and avoid a "laboratory error" will be a great service in saving both time and money, as well as possibly saving the patient from a needless venipuncture.

Review Questions

1. Probably the most important aspect of phlebotomy is proper _____.
2. The cleanser of choice for routine venipuncture is _____.
3. The _____ should always be released before removing the needle from a vein.
4. You should always _____ before moving on to the next patient.
5. _____ may cause an elevation in blood enzymes.

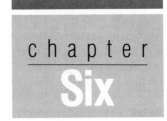

chapter
Six

Special Collection Procedures

John C. Flynn, Jr.

A well-trained and experienced phlebotomist is a valuable asset to the clinical laboratory. Often the phlebotomist is asked or required to do more than perform routine venipunctures or microcapillary collections. This chapter outlines other blood collection procedures or tests that phlebotomists may perform depending on the institution where they are employed.

BLEEDING TIME TEST

A bleeding time test is a rather simple test that is used to ascertain the functioning of a patient's platelets. Platelets are crucial in stopping capillary bleeding, and the bleeding time gives the clinician information about the integrity of the patient's platelet function. A prolonged bleed-

87

ing time indicates that either the platelet count is low or the platelets are not functioning properly.

Although it is not the responsibility of phlebotomists to monitor the medications a patient may be taking, they should be aware that certain drugs will prolong the bleeding time. The most noteworthy among these drugs are aspirin and aspirin-containing compounds. Aspirin impairs platelets' ability to form aggregates. Antihistamines also interfere with bleeding time.

The Ivy method is the most popular procedure to determine bleeding time. This involves applying a sphygmomanometer (blood pressure) cuff to the upper arm and inflating it to 40 mm Hg. After the volar area of the arm is cleansed with 70% isopropyl alcohol, two small incisions are made with a commercially available, standardized instrument (Fig. 6–1A,B). Then every 30 seconds the blood is blotted, not wiped, with filter paper until bleeding is stopped (Fig. 6–1C), at which time the sphygmomanometer cuff can be released. The difference between the two sites should not be more than 30 seconds. If bleeding occurs for more than 15 minutes, the cuff is released, and the results are noted simply as greater than 15 minutes. The phlebotomist should remain with the patient until bleeding stops. The results are recorded and returned to the laboratory.

NEONATAL BLOOD COLLECTION

With the increasing sophistication of medical testing and care, premature infants have a better chance of survival today than they did as recently as 1980. Infants as small as 2 lb or less in weight and more than 10 weeks premature are surviving. To monitor the progress of care and treatment, blood must be collected for analysis.

Collecting blood from infants involves using a variation of the microcollection techniques previously discussed in Chapter 5. The site of collection is generally the infant's foot. Care must be exercised when performing the skin puncture to avoid damaging the heel bone, which can cause **osteomyelitis** in the newborn. Figure 6–2A illustrates the safe areas to perform the puncture.

When preparing to perform the blood collection, take only the equipment necessary into the bassinet area to avoid needlessly exposing a generally weakened infant to additional bacteria. You will usually be required to wear at least a gown in addition to gloves. Try not to disturb the infant any more than necessary, and if you must change the infant's position, do so only with permission of the nurse because of the many tubes and lines that are often attached to premature infants. Prepare the puncture site as described in Chapter 5, and hold the heel firmly as

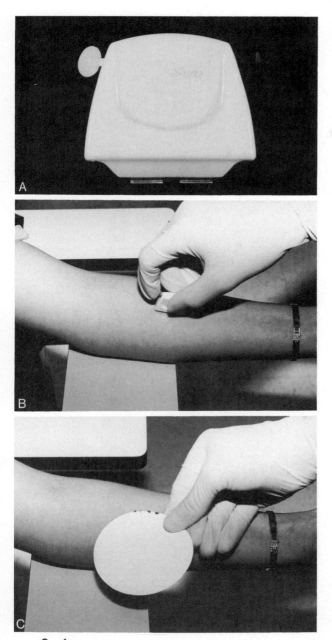

figure **6-1** *A,* Commercial bleeding time instrument. *B,* Making the incisions. *C,* Blotting the incisions with filter paper.

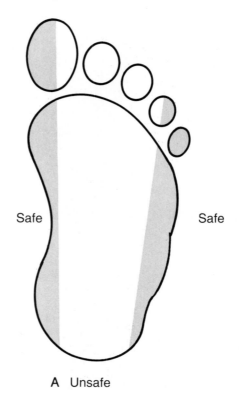

A Unsafe

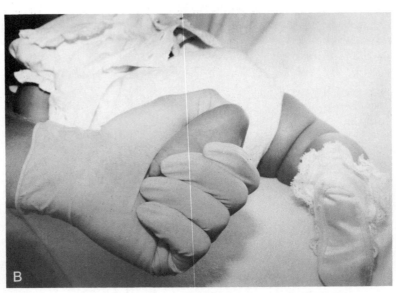

figure **6-2**   *A,* Safe areas on an infant's foot for microcapillary collection. *B,* A properly held heel for skin puncture.

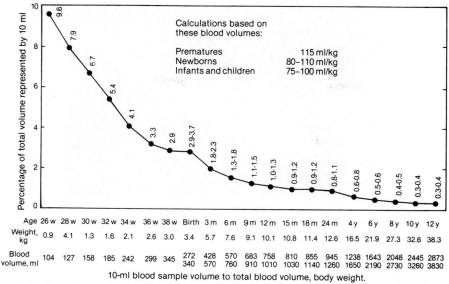

Calculations based on these blood volumes:

Prematures	115 ml/kg
Newborns	80–110 ml/kg
Infants and children	75–100 ml/kg

Age	26 w	28 w	30 w	32 w	34 w	36 w	38 w	Birth	3 m	6 m	9 m	12 m	15 m	18 m	24 m	4 y	6 y	8 y	10 y	12 y
Weight, kg	0.9	4.1	1.3	1.6	2.1	2.6	3.0	3.4	5.7	7.6	9.1	10.1	10.8	11.4	12.6	16.5	21.9	27.3	32.6	38.3
Blood volume, ml	104	127	158	185	242	299	345	272 340	428 570	570 760	683 910	758 1010	810 1030	855 1140	945 1260	1238 1650	1643 2190	2048 2730	2445 3260	2873 3830

10-ml blood sample volume to total blood volume, body weight.

figure **6–3** Relationship of 10-ml blood sample to total blood volume, body weight, and age of patient. (From Slockbower JM, Blumenfeld TA, eds: Collection and Handling of Laboratory Specimens. Philadelphia, JB Lippincott, 1983.)

shown in Figure 6–2*B*. Perform the skin puncture and wipe away the first drop of blood. Collect blood into the appropriate container, being careful not to apply too much pressure to the heel; this could adversely affect the results of testing, as well as hurt the infant. When you are finished, apply pressure until bleeding has stopped. *Do not apply a bandage, and do not leave anything in the bassinet.* Label the collected specimens appropriately and deliver them to the laboratory.

Because of the small total blood volume of newborns (Fig. 6–3), a log should be kept of the total blood removed from infants. Often anemia becomes a problem because of the amount of blood collected from a given newborn. Therefore, accurate records must be maintained.

SYRINGE COLLECTIONS

At one time a syringe was the only option for blood collection. With the advent of the evacuated tube system, the use of a syringe to collect venous blood is no longer even routine. Generally, a syringe is used to collect blood from veins that may collapse when using an evacuated tube system (e.g., small or fragile veins often found in elderly patients and small children). See Figure 6–4 for an illustration of a typical syringe.

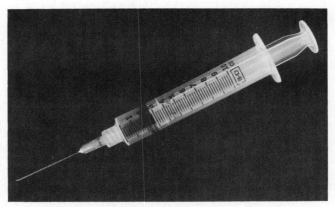

figure **6-4**   A typical syringe.

Collecting blood via the syringe is really rather simple. Preparation of the venipuncture site is the same as that for the evacuated tube system described in Chapter 5. However, use of the syringe does differ significantly from that of the evacuated tube system in the order in which the tubes are filled once the blood is collected in the syringe. Because blood will begin to clot in the syringe, it is imperative that collected blood be added to the anticoagulant tubes (i.e., the sodium citrate [blue-stoppered] tubes) first, followed by any other anticoagulant tubes, and then any remaining tubes without anticoagulant. The phlebotomist should mix the anticoagulant tubes thoroughly after the blood has been added, and it is advisable to carefully remove the syringe needle to facilitate the addition of blood to the tubes. Figure 6-5 illustrates the order for tube filling.

GLUCOSE TOLERANCE TEST

The glucose tolerance test (GTT) is done on individuals who are being screened for **diabetes mellitus** or **hypoglycemia.** Although there is nothing unique about the actual collection process itself, the number of venipunctures performed in a relatively short period of time make this test significant. The purpose of the test is to determine the patient's blood glucose level after the patient consumes a fixed amount of glucose (usually 100 gm). The test takes from 3 to 5 hours.

After a patient has fasted for at least 12 hours, a blood sample is collected using routine collection procedures. The blood may be collected in a plain tube (without any anticoagulant) or in a tube especially de-

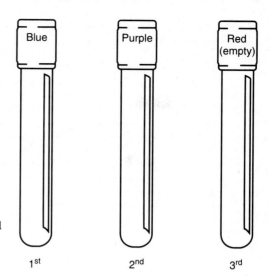

figure **6-5**

Proper order for filling tubes with blood collected via syringe. Sodium citrate anticoagulant tubes (blue-stoppered) must be filled first, followed by any other anticoagulant tubes and then any remaining tubes without anticoagulant.

signed to preserve glucose levels (e.g., gray-stoppered tubes with sodium fluoride and potassium oxalate).

After the fasting sample is collected, the patient is directed to consume 100 gm of glucose as quickly as possible, often in liquid form. *It is critical to note the time of glucose consumption and of all subsequent venipunctures.* Blood is then collected at ½ hour, 1 hour, 2 hours, 3 hours, etc., up to 5 hours after consuming the glucose. At each venipuncture a urine specimen is also collected. Again, it is very important to note the collection time on all specimens.

The laboratory analyzes the glucose levels in the blood specimens and plots them on a chart (Fig. 6-6). The results help the physician determine whether the patient is suffering from diabetes.

The phlebotomist plays a very crucial role in the administration of this test. Usually the patient receives a set of instructions about what to eat and a warning to avoid stressful exercise in the days leading up to the GTT. However, it is often the phlebotomist who gives the patient instructions about dieting and fasting. The patient should eat a well-balanced diet for 3 days before the test. Generally, the patient is allowed water and is actually encouraged to drink water during the fast and the test, but nothing else is allowed, including coffee and tea. Smoking is also discouraged. These instructions must be delivered in a clear and understandable manner. Patients should be encouraged to ask questions if they do not understand the instructions. If the phlebotomist does not perform

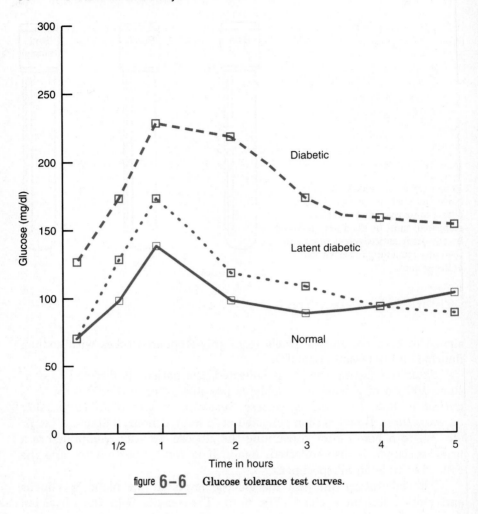

figure **6-6**   Glucose tolerance test curves.

this patient education function properly, much valuable time may be wasted.

Finally, the phlebotomist must be prepared to handle the situation when the patient becomes ill from consuming the glucose or "light-headed" from fasting for several hours. Generally, nausea and vomiting occur early in the test, and it is a good idea to have towels and an emesis basin nearby. If the patient vomits within the first ½ hour, the test should be discontinued and will probably need to be rescheduled for another day. If the patient vomits or becomes faint later in the test, have him or her lie down, and complete the testing. If repeated oral glucose administrations are unsuccessful, intravenously administered glucose is an option. The patient's physician will make this decision.

ARTERIAL PUNCTURES

Although they are *very infrequently* performed by phlebotomists, arterial punctures should be mentioned. Generally, a nurse or respiratory therapist will collect an arterial blood specimen to assay for blood gases. The blood gas determination reveals, among other things, how well the lungs are functioning in terms of gas exchange. It should be clearly explained to the patient that this procedure is more uncomfortable than venipuncture and more difficult to accomplish.

The obvious difference between the arterial puncture and the venipuncture is the blood vessel from which the specimen is collected. The artery of choice is often the brachial artery, which is located on the inside of the upper arm (Fig. 6-7). It can be found by feeling for a pulse using the middle finger and forefinger; the thumb is not used because its pulse may be confused with that of the artery. A second possible site is the arteries found in the wrist area.

The puncture site should be cleansed with a provodine-iodine (Betadine) solution. No tourniquet is needed because of the pressure that already exists within the arteries. A syringe may be used, since generally only a small amount of blood (1 ml) is needed. The syringe should be capped, placed in ice, and transported to the laboratory as soon as possible after collection. Ideally, the test should be run within 10 minutes after collection.

The phlebotomist should maintain pressure on the site for at least 15 minutes after collection. It takes much longer for bleeding to stop in an artery than in a vein. The patient should never be allowed to maintain pressure, and the patient's nurse should be made aware that an arterial puncture was done so that she or he can periodically check the puncture site.

COLD AGGLUTININ TESTS

A cold agglutinin is an antibody that is made in response to a form of pneumonia called primary atypical pneumonia, which is caused by the bacteria *Mycoplasma pneumoniae.* Therefore, the presence of a cold agglutinin is diagnostic. Occasionally the antibody can cause a form of autoimmune hemolytic anemia.

The key to collection of a specimen that will be screened for cold agglutinins is maintaining the specimen at 37°C after collection. The

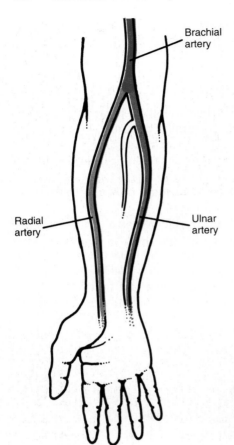

figure **6-7**

The brachial artery is the preferred site for arterial puncture. A wrist artery may also be used.

specimen is collected in an empty evacuated tube (plain red stopper) after proper site preparation and delivered promptly to the laboratory, where it is placed in a 37°C incubator. If prompt delivery is not possible, the specimen may be placed in a temporary holding device such as a cup of water that is 37°C. The water must not be warmer than 37°C, as this may alter the test result. Similarly, should the specimen be allowed to cool, the results may be invalid.

BLOOD CULTURES

Under normal conditions, blood is a sterile substance. When bacteria enter into the bloodstream, this condition is referred to as **septicemia.** Septicemia is a very serious condition and must be detected and treated as soon as possible. Because blood circulates throughout the body, bacteria in the blood can be transported to other areas of the body, thereby spreading infection. The proper antibiotics must be administered to stop the infection.

To administer the proper antibiotics, the offending bacteria must be identified. To do this, a blood culture must be performed. The phlebotomist's role is to collect a specimen using special sterilization techniques.

One symptom of septicemia is a fever of unknown origin (FUO). Often such a fever will rise and fall on a regular basis. Therefore, timing of the blood culture is crucial. It is often desirable to collect blood cultures before and after a fever "spikes." This maximizes the chances of collecting a specimen while the bacteria is present in the bloodstream.

After a vein is located, the site is specially prepared for venipuncture. With the tourniquet off, the site is thoroughly scrubbed using surgical green soap for 2 minutes. A sterile alcohol pad is used to remove the soap by rubbing in outward-moving concentric circles (Fig. 6–8). The alcohol must be allowed to air dry. The site is then cleaned with a povidone-iodine solution, which is also allowed to air dry. The tourniquet is applied, and the venipuncture is performed. The site can be touched only with sterile gauze or with a finger that has been cleaned in the same way used for the site.

Although some aspects of blood culture collection will vary from institution to institution, all techniques involve collecting blood either directly or indirectly into an **aerobic** and **anaerobic** culture system. Either a syringe or a specially designed evacuated tube is used (Fig. 6–9A). When a syringe is used, a clean needle is placed on the syringe after blood collection, and then the blood culture bottles are inoculated (anaerobic followed by aerobic).

The blood may also be collected into an evacuated tube made especially for blood cultures; then, in the laboratory, a syringe is used to remove blood from the evacuated tube and inoculate the blood culture

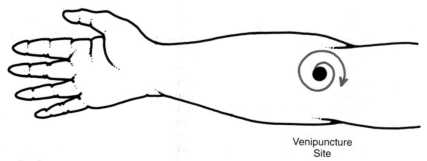

Venipuncture
Site

figure **6–8**   Proper method for swabbing a venipuncture site, moving in an outward spiral.

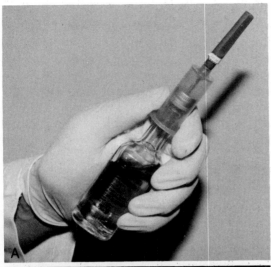

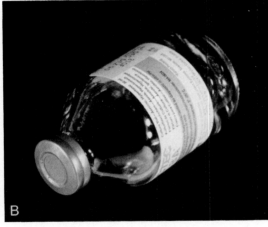

figure **6–9**

Examples of culture systems used in collection of blood cultures. *A*, Specially designed Vacutainer tube for collecting a blood culture (direct method). *B*, Typical blood culture bottle (indirect method).

bottles (Fig. 6–9*B*). However, no matter what collection method is used, care must be taken to maintain sterility by swabbing the septum of the culture bottles with iodine followed by alcohol.

After the blood is collected, the povidone-iodine solution can be removed using alcohol swabs. The culture bottles must be thoroughly mixed and labeled with pertinent information, including the time and site of collection. This is important, because blood cultures are collected rather frequently, and the policy at some hospitals is to alternate arms at each blood culture collection.

BLOOD DONATION COLLECTIONS

Phlebotomists may be employed in a blood donation center, where they collect blood that will ultimately be used for transfusion. These centers may be American Red Cross Centers, Community Blood Center, or hospital blood banks and collection centers.

Phlebotomists who collect blood from volunteer donors must be very competent in the skill of venipuncture and must possess good interpersonal skills. Because relatively few individuals (less than 5% of the population) provide donor blood for the entire country, it is very critical that every phase of the donation process be performed smoothly and professionally. The health care system cannot afford the loss of these volunteer donors, and an unpleasant experience may discourage them from volunteering again.

This type of blood collection varies from routine venipuncture in two ways: the amount of blood that is collected (usually 450 ml) and the nature of the "patient." Individuals who donate blood must undergo a thorough medical history and screening. The history should include frequency of donation, present and past medications, exposure to transfusion-transmitted disease such as hepatitis B and human immunodeficiency virus (HIV), recent vaccinations, foreign travel, and cancer history. The medical screening includes monitoring blood pressure, temperature, hemoglobin or hematocrit, weight, pulse, skin lesions, and general appearance. Donors also complete a donor self-exclusion form, which allows them to confidentially ensure that their blood will not be used for transfusion if they have any misgivings. The American Association of Blood Banks' *Technical Manual* contains a more thorough discussion of donor criteria. Once the donor passes the medical history and screening, the actual phlebotomy can be performed. The antecubital area of the arm is the preferred site and must be thoroughly cleaned and disinfected. (See the procedure discussed earlier for blood culture preparation.) The step-by-step procedure for performing blood donor phlebotomy is as follows:

1. Once the donor is comfortably situated — generally on a bed or special donor chair — locate the vein.
2. Prepare the site.
3. Prepare the blood collection bag and scale. Be sure there is a clamp between the bag and the needle.
4. Apply the tourniquet or blood pressure cuff (inflated to 40 to 60 mm Hg), and give the donor something to squeeze. These techniques will help distend the vein.
5. Perform the venipuncture and place the needle approximately ½ inch into the vein.

6. Release the clamp; if there is a steady flow of blood into the bag, tape the needle to the arm. Cover the area with sterile gauze.

7. Release the tourniquet or blood pressure cuff, but instruct the donor to clench his or her fist. Monitor the donor for any adverse reactions. (These are infrequent; see Chapter 7.)

8. When the appropriate volume of blood (405 to 450 ml) is collected, instruct the donor to stop clenching the fist, and clamp or tie a knot in the tubing.

9. Collect pilot tubes — samples of donor blood that will be tested before the unit is released for transfusion — before removing the needle from the donor's arm.

10. Strip the tubing and thoroughly mix the blood; then allow the tubing to refill. At this time the tubing may be segmented.

11. Place the units in storage as specified by the collection room nurse or technologist.

12. Do not allow the patient to arise or leave the area until bleeding has stopped and at least 10 minutes have elapsed. Because the donor has lost a significant amount of blood, be sure to instruct him or her to increase fluid intake over the next 24 hours, avoid alcohol until after a meal, avoid smoking for at least 30 minutes, refrain from strenuous exercise for a few hours, apply pressure if bleeding resumes, and sit down if dizziness occurs. They may have to return to the blood bank or see their own doctor if symptoms continue.

13. Finally, *always be polite and professional.* The donor should leave with a positive feeling so that he or she will be inclined to donate blood again.

THERAPEUTIC COLLECTIONS

As mentioned in Chapter 1, in ancient times, therapeutic phlebotomy was the only treatment used for many different conditions. Today the treatment is used very judiciously. Blood is collected as an aid to treatment of some diseases such as **polycythemia vera** or **myasthenia gravis.** It is rarely the definitive treatment, but instead serves as symptomatic treatment until the underlying cause can be identified and treated.

Therapeutic phlebotomies are very similar to donor blood collection, but the underlying purpose is different. Whereas donated blood is destined to be used for transfusion, blood collected for a therapeutic reason is generally discarded or occasionally is used for research purposes. Therefore, no additional pilot tubes of blood need be collected for additional testing. In addition, the amount of blood collected may be different; an amount less than 450 ml may be appropriate depending on the patient's age and condition. However, site preparation is the same, and the same precautions must be observed when performing therapeutic phlebotomies.

TESTS FOR FIBRIN DEGRADATION PRODUCTS

Fibrin degradation products (FDPs) are the result of the disintegration of fibrin or fibrinogen by plasmin, a coagulation enzyme. Increased levels of FDPs are generally associated with such conditions as myocardial infarctions, pulmonary emboli, certain complications of pregnancy, and disseminated intravascular coagulation.

A popular test for detecting FDPs is the Thrombo-Wellcotest (Burroughs-Wellcome, Triangle Park, NC). For the phlebotomist, this test involves performing a routine venipuncture using a tube provided with the test kit. The tube will hold 2 ml of blood and contains a special enzyme inhibitor plus thrombin. It is important to avoid traumatic venipunctures that might result in hemolysis, and the sample must be gently but thoroughly mixed after collection.

Once the sample is collected, assays are performed in the laboratory to semiquantitate the FDPs. This information is important to the clinician in making the proper diagnosis. Occasionally, urine may be tested for FDPs.

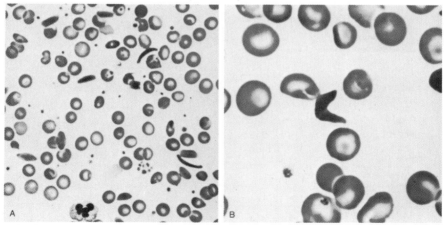

figure **6-10** Blood smear from a patient with sickle cell anemia. *A*, Low magnification shows sickled cells. *B*, Higher magnification shows an irreversibly sickled cell in the center. (Courtesy of Dr. Robert W. McKenna, University of Texas, Southwestern Medical School, Dallas, TX.)

PERIPHERAL BLOOD SMEARS

Peripheral blood smears are important to the clinician for a number of reasons. Examination of the blood smear may reveal abnormal red cell morphology characteristic of certain disease states such as sickle cell anemia (Fig. 6–10). The variety and proportion of white blood cells may also be ascertained; information of this nature may also help in the

1. Place slide on flat surface;
   Apply drop of blood.

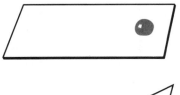

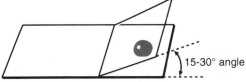

15-30° angle

2. Immediately bring "spreader"
   slide back to drop.

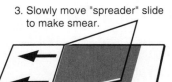

3. Slowly move "spreader" slide
   to make smear.

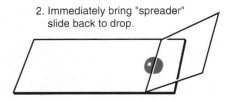

Feather edge

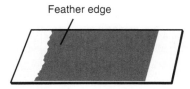

figure **6–11**

"Wedge" method, the suggested method for making blood smears.

diagnosis of disease. For example, infectious mononucleosis is characterized by an increased number of "atypical" lymphocytes.

Although the process is becoming increasingly semiautomated, phlebotomists may still be called on to make a blood smear. This may be
done either at the patient's bedside using standard microscope slides and
capillary blood or in the laboratory using well-mixed, recently collected
(within 1 hour) anticoagulated (with ethylenediaminetetra-acetate) blood.

The "wedge" method is probably the most common manual method
(Fig. 6–11). The following important points should be remembered:

Keep the smear slide on a flat surface.
Make the smear immediately after placing the blood on the slide.
Make the smear in a smooth fashion to avoid ridges and bubbles.
Allow the smear to air dry; never blow on it.
A straight-edge smear is preferable to a bullet-shaped smear because of
    better distribution of leukocytes.

It takes a great deal of practice to become proficient at making
smears, and therefore it may be desirable to assign slide making to
certain members of the phlebotomy team.

chapter
Six
Review
Questions

1. Arterial puncture is the method of choice for _____.
2. The volume of blood usually collected during blood donation is
   _____.
3. Bacteria in the blood is referred to as _____.
4. _____ is an infection of the bone that may be caused by penetra-
   tion of the heel bone with a lancet.
5. The device inflated to 40 mm Hg when a phlebotomist is performing the Ivy bleeding time test is a _____.

Bibliography

Goss CM, ed. Gray's Anatomy: Anatomy of the Human Body. 28th ed. Philadelphia, Lea &
    Febiger, 1966.
Harmening DM, ed. Clinical Hematology and Fundamentals of Hemostasis. 2nd ed. Phila-
    delphia, FA Davis, 1992.

Nursing79 Books. Managing Diabetics Properly. Horsham, PA, Intermed Communications Inc., 1978.

Slockbower JM, Blumenfeld TA, eds. Collection and Handling of Laboratory Specimens. Philadelphia, JB Lippincott, 1983.

Tietz NW, ed. Fundamentals of Clinical Chemistry. 3rd ed. Philadelphia, WB Saunders, 1987.

Walker RH, ed. Technical Manual. 10th ed. Arlington, VA, American Association of Blood Banks, 1990.

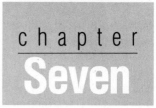

Complications of Phlebotomy

John C. Flynn, Jr.

This chapter will discuss various complications that can be encountered while performing or attempting to perform phlebotomy. These include uncooperative or absent patients, medical/physiologic complications, and technical problems.

THE UNCOOPERATIVE PATIENT

Every phlebotomist has encountered an uncooperative patient. The patient may be uncooperative for a variety of reasons (e.g., age [young or old], which may preclude him or her from understanding the procedure; there may be mental dysfunction; or the patient may object to having the phlebotomy done for some other reason).

When a patient is too old or young to understand what is going on and will probably resist or struggle, do not attempt to perform the venipuncture alone. Get help from the patient's nurse, a fellow phlebotomist, or a parent, relative, or guardian. Take precautions to ensure the safety

105

of the individual, but do not compromise your own safety. A common and safe way to hold a child is shown in Figure 7-1.

Occasionally phlebotomists are required to collect blood from a patient who is mentally disturbed, mentally retarded, or suffering from substance abuse. In such a case, the patient may not understand the procedure and may react violently. You must do what you can to reassure the patient and secure cooperation. However, if there is any doubt about how the patient will react, do not attempt to collect the specimen until you have secured some assistance, even if the patient is in restraints.

Sometimes a patient may be of sound mind and yet still refuse to have the procedure performed. At these times you must use your skills of persuasion to convince the patient to allow you to collect the blood sample. Point out that the physician needs the blood test results to properly manage the patient's illness and prescribe the proper medication. Never attempt to force, either physically or with threats, a patient in this situation. Ultimately, if the patient refuses to allow the blood collection, this must be noted on the requisition form, which is returned to the laboratory; the patient's nurse must also be informed.

Another situation that often confronts a phlebotomist is that of an absent patient — that is, the patient is not where he or she is supposed to be. The patient may have been moved to another room or transported to

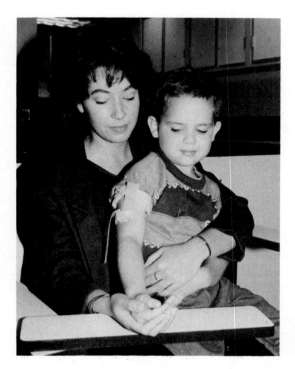

figure **7-1**

A suggested way to restrain a child for phlebotomy.

surgery or the radiology department. He or she may have been discharged or perhaps may have **expired.** Generally, the phlebotomist can find out where the patient is by asking the nurse in charge. If the patient has simply been moved to another room, collect the blood specimen, noting the room change on the requisition form and on the tube of blood. If the patient is inaccessible (e.g., in radiology or the operating room), inform the patient's nurse and note on the requisition form why the blood was not collected.

MEDICAL/PHYSIOLOGIC COMPLICATIONS

Common Complications

SYNCOPE

Syncope, more commonly referred to as fainting, results from insufficient blood flow to the brain. This can be caused by fatigue, a sudden decrease in blood volume, cardiac arrhythmia, hypoglycemia, or hyperventilation. However, fainting is primarily due to psychological causes in individuals who are having their blood collected. Merely the sight of blood or needles is enough to cause some people to faint.

To prevent fainting or to deal effectively with it, the phlebotomist must always be aware of the condition of the patient. Observe the patient before the phlebotomy; is he or she acting nervous or hyperventilating? Try to engage the patient in conversation to keep his or her mind off the procedure. After performing the venipuncture, ask the patient how he or she feels.

Whereas the volume of blood collected during routine phlebotomy is not enough in itself to cause fainting due to **hypovolemia,** hypovolemia may cause fainting in blood donation. As stated in Chapter 6, blood donation results in about a 450-ml loss of blood from the donor. This loss may be enough to cause syncope if the patient attempts to get out of the donor chair too quickly. This is why the donor is not allowed to leave the chair for at least 10 minutes after the collection. This time, along with the consumption of some liquids, gives the body a chance to adjust to the decreased total blood volume.

If a patient is sitting in a chair and faints before the venipuncture, put the patient's head between his or her knees (Fig. 7–2). A cold compress placed on the back of the neck is also helpful. It is also a good idea to have ammonium salts available, but these can be very strong and must be used with care. Once the patient recovers, have him or her lie down for the phlebotomy to be performed. A cool drink may also help the patient feel better. Patients who are lying down very seldom feel faint. If

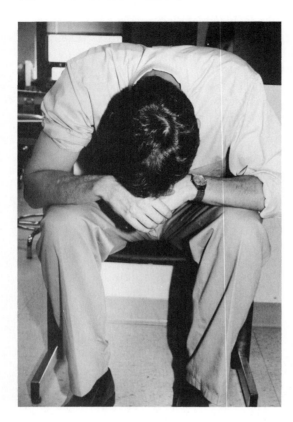

figure **7–2**

If the patient feels faint, place the head between the knees.

the patient feels faint after the phlebotomy has been started, remove the tourniquet, carefully remove the needle, and, while applying pressure, support the patient and call for help. *Never leave the patient!*

HEMATOMA

Probably the most common complication from phlebotomy is the **hematoma.** This occurs when the needle is improperly placed in the vein, allowing blood to escape from the vein and collect under the skin (Fig. 7–3). The primary indication of a hematoma is swelling around the venipuncture site while the needle is inserted. By adjusting the depth of the needle, it may be possible to stop the hematoma from enlarging. Otherwise, the best thing to do is remove the needle and apply firm pressure to the site. This may help the blood to disperse somewhat. It is usually good practice and common courtesy to inform the patient that he or she may notice a bruise in a day or two at the venipuncture site. It is nothing to be alarmed about and will disappear in a few days.

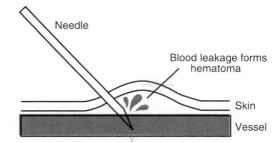

figure **7-3**

A hematoma occurs when an improperly placed needle causes blood to escape from the vein.

If removal of the needle is required and not enough blood was collected, another venipuncture must be performed. This venipuncture should be at an alternate site.

SHORT DRAW OR NO BLOOD COLLECTED

Occasionally, the phlebotomist will enter the vein, and the blood flow will be slow or will stop after a short time, or blood will not flow at all. There are some general technical errors that can occur; these are discussed later. There are also some occasions when the needle is in the vein, but blood flow is reduced. In such cases, the needle bevel may be against the vessel wall (Fig. 7-4A), thus preventing the flow of blood. Slight manipulation of the needle will generally remedy this problem. In other cases the suction of the vacuum may be too great, causing the vessel to collapse (Fig. 7-4B). In these cases smaller tubes or a syringe may be used to collect the blood. Collapsed veins may also occur if the syringe plunger is withdrawn too quickly.

Less Common Complications

Petechiae. Petechiae are small red dots that appear on the skin as the result of capillary **hemorrhage.** In such cases, the capillaries bleed excessively because of a coagulation problem, generally one related to platelets. As stated in Chapter 2, the function of platelets is to stop bleeding from blood vessel walls. If you notice petechiae, you should realize that it may take a little longer than normal for the patient to stop bleeding from the venipuncture site. Petechiae can also be the result of tying the tourniquet too tight and leaving it on too long. For this reason the tourniquet should not be on for longer than 1 to 2 minutes.

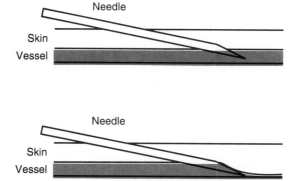

figure **7-4**

Two possible causes of a "short draw," or failure to obtain blood. *A*, The needle bevel is against the vessel wall, preventing blood flow. *B*, The vacuum causes the vessel to collapse.

Edema. **Edema** results when excessive fluids collect in the tissues of a patient, resulting in swelling. Venipuncture should be avoided in these areas, because (1) it is often difficult to locate a vein, and (2) the specimen may be diluted with tissue fluids, which could adversely affect the testing results.

Obesity. Locating and palpating a vein may be difficult in an obese patient, as the veins are generally "deeper" and cannot be seen. However, with practice and patience, you will learn to locate these veins and perform the phlebotomy with minimal difficulty.

Allergies. Occasionally patients may indicate that they are allergic to a sterilizing solution or to the adhesive on bandages. When a patient expresses these concerns, the phlebotomist should find an alternative.

Damaged or Scarred Veins. Occasionally you will encounter a patient who has had so many venipunctures that an area of scar tissue has developed around the area that you plan to use for phlebotomy. For example, it is not unusual for intravenous drug users to have a lot of scar tissue. These situations require an alternative site for venipuncture, and if none can be located (which would be unusual), a microcapillary procedure should be considered. Veins may also be damaged or occluded (blocked) to the degree that even if the venipuncture is successful, little blood is collected. Again, an alternate site must be located.

Burned Areas. Burned areas must be avoided altogether, as they are very susceptible to infection. The phlebotomist must take extra precautions when performing venipuncture on these patients. Gowns and face masks are required, because the patient is at risk of contracting an infection from the phlebotomist (see Chapter 3). An alternate site for venipuncture must be chosen or a microcollection technique utilized.

Convulsions. Although **convulsions** resulting from phlebotomy are rare, a phlebotomist must be prepared to deal with them. It is a good practice to ask patients if they have had any previous adverse reactions to phlebotomy. Although many things can cause convulsions, simple hysteria causes most convulsions in phlebotomy patients. The most important thing is to not let patients harm themselves. If the needle is in the arm, quickly remove it and the tourniquet, if the latter is still on the arm. Move anything that could harm the patient and try to protect the patient's head from striking an object that could cause harm. Do not forget to call for help and notify a physician. If the patient is in a chair and starts to fall out, help guide him or her to the floor. *Do not panic, and never leave the patient alone!* Be sure to record the date, time, and circumstances under which the convulsion occurred. Once the patient recovers, assess the situation to determine whether the phlebotomy can be done or repeated, if required, or whether the patient should return at a later time.

TECHNICAL PROBLEMS

The technical problems discussed in this section include situations that result in no blood being collected because of either faulty equipment or simply missing the vein. Occasionally everything is done properly, but when the tube is pushed onto the needle, no blood is forthcoming. This could be due to a faulty collection tube that does not contain any vacuum or because the phlebotomist unknowingly pushed the tube onto the needle during the process of preparing to perform the venipuncture, thus releasing the vacuum. It is always a good practice to carry extra collection tubes and keep them within easy reach whenever performing a phlebotomy.

Another technical problem that occasionally occurs is having the needle unscrew from the barrel during the phlebotomy. If this occurs, do not attempt to correct the problem; simply discontinue the phlebotomy, and repeat the procedure. Make sure that the needle is properly seated in the hub of the barrel so that the problem does not happen again.

All phlebotomists, at some point in their career, will miss the target vein completely. When this occurs, it may be possible to simply redirect the needle slightly and obtain blood. You may be to one side of the vein or perhaps did not enter the needle deep enough. *However, avoid probing!*

The more experience you get as a phlebotomist, the less frequently you will miss, and when you do, it will be easier for you to redirect the needle without having to repeat the entire venipuncture procedure.

SPECIMEN REJECTION

This section will outline some of the common reasons why specimens may be rejected by the clinical laboratory.

Hemolysis

Hemolysis occurs when red blood cells are destroyed, thus releasing a red-tinted substance, hemoglobin. Hemolysis may not be evident at the time of collection but becomes evident in the laboratory when the specimens are centrifuged to separate the cells from the serum or plasma. Depending on the test being performed, a hemolyzed specimen may not be acceptable. For example, hemolysis may interfere with testing done in the blood bank. In other areas, the hemolysis or hemoglobin itself may not be a problem, but other constituents released when the cells were destroyed may interfere with testing or give falsely high or low values. See Table 7–1 for some common tests and the effect hemolysis may have on them.

Hemolysis may be a result of a physiologic condition, such as autoimmune hemolytic anemia or a transfusion reaction, that causes hemoglobin to be present in the patient's plasma. More often it is a result of the venipuncture procedure itself or the handling of the specimen after

table **7–1**   THE EFFECTS OF HEMOLYSIS ON COMMON TESTS

Test	Effect
Chemistry	
Potassium	Increased value
Magnesium	Increased value
Aldolase	Increased value
Lactate dehydrogenase	Increased value
Blood bank	
Antibody screen	May invalidate test; specimen rejected
Hematology	
Prothrombin time	Increased value if severe
Activated partial thromboplastin time	Increased value if severe

table **7-2**	CAUSES OF HEMOLYSIS

Technical
　　Vigorously shaking the tube of blood
　　Using a needle that is too small
　　Drawing too hard on the syringe plunger
　　Expelling blood too quickly through the syringe into the collection tubes
　　Allowing the specimen to overheat
Physiologic
　　Transfusion reaction
　　Autoimmune hemolytic anemia
　　Paroxysmal nocturnal hemoglobinuria
　　Disseminated intravascular coagulation

collection. See Table 7-2 for a list of items that may result when a specimen is hemolyzed.

If the phlebotomist follows standard procedures and is conscientious, most cases of phlebotomy-induced hemolysis can be avoided. This in turn will save time, money, and, most important, the need to perform a repeat phlebotomy on the patient.

Clots

Clot formation occurs when **coagulation factors** are activated. Normally, if no anticoagulants are present in the collection tube, these factors are activated almost immediately. When a clot forms in an anticoagulant specimen, generally the specimen will be rejected and a new one will have to be collected. When a clot begins to form in an anticoagulated tube, it usually indicates that the blood and anticoagulant are not in proper balance. If too little blood is collected, or if too much blood is added to an anticoagulant tube — as, for example, via a syringe — a clot may form. Therefore, whenever using an evacuated tube system, always fill the tube with the amount of blood indicated.

Clots may also be present when blood is collected into a syringe and not expelled soon enough into an anticoagulant tube. For this reason blood collected via a syringe is expressed into an anticoagulant tube, rather than an empty tube, first.

Finally, clots may form because the anticoagulant itself is not active or is not present in the proper quantity. The phlebotomist may not be aware of this, and therefore, it is very important to check the expiration date on the tubes. As long as they are in date, everything should be acceptable.

Short Draw

A short draw is a specimen that does not contain enough blood. Depending on the tests being performed, a short draw may result in specimen rejection. A short draw may occur when the needle comes out of the vein, when the vein collapses, or when the vacuum was not sufficient to fill the tube. If the vein collapses, you will probably have to redraw the specimen from a different site or possibly use a syringe. If the needle came out of the vein and you can reinsert it, you will avoid a short draw. Otherwise the venipuncture may need to be repeated. Possibly the vacuum was not strong enough; in this case, the extra tubes you should be carrying will enable you collect the specimen without needing to "restick" the patient.

Clerical Discrepancies

Clerical discrepancies occur when the name on the requisition form does not match the name on the tube of blood. Depending on the institution and the laboratory department, there will be variations in how clerical discrepancies are handled. For example, a specimen with a slightly misspelled patient name may be acceptable for hematology if the patient's hospital number, room number, etc., are correct. However, for transfusion units or blood banks, which have the strictest requirements, the slightest deviation in name or hospital number may require collection of a new specimen. The reason should be obvious: a transfusion based on the results of an incorrectly labeled specimen could be fatal!

chapter **Seven** # Review Questions

1. Small red dots on the skin indicating a possible coagulation problem are _____.
2. Low blood volume is referred to as _____.
3. _____ is a condition in which fluid collects in the tissues and results in swelling.
4. _____ is the destruction of red blood cells that results in the release of hemoglobin.
5. Blood that escapes from a blood vessel and collects under the skin may result in a _____.

Bibliography

Thomas CL, ed. Taber's Cyclopedic Medical Dictionary. 16th ed. Philadelphia, FA Davis, 1989.

Tietz NW, ed. Fundamentals of Clinical Chemistry. 3rd ed. Philadelphia, WB Saunders, 1987.

Walker RH, ed. Technical Manual. 10th ed. Arlington, VA, American Association of Blood Banks, 1990.

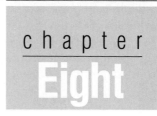
Animal Phlebotomy

Beth V. Dronson

The purpose of this chapter is to acquaint laboratory personnel and students with basic knowledge of animal venipuncture, blood handling techniques, and common tests performed on animals. Often the most difficult part of animal venipuncture is patient cooperation, so the first section explains animal restraint and various venipuncture sites. The major laboratory species of dog, cat, rabbit, rat, mouse, and guinea pig are included in the discussion. The second section explores proper blood handling techniques, including the effects produced by hemolysis and **lipemia.** Appendix tables at the end of the chapter cover common tests run on laboratory animals as well as the types of tube used and the size sample needed.

TECHNIQUES FOR OBTAINING BLOOD SAMPLES FROM ANIMALS

The major laboratory species (dog, cat, rabbit, rat, mouse, and guinea pig) each require different venipuncture techniques. In each species there are multiple sites available for venipuncture depending on the amount of blood needed and the type of testing to be done. Each site requires a different restraint technique, often involving an assistant. However, certain general guidelines apply to all species.

General Guidelines for Animal Venipuncture

1. Animals should be handled gently and spoken to softly. It is much easier to handle and to obtain samples from a calm animal. In addition, stress should be avoided, because it can lead to biochemical changes in the blood that are not indicative of physiologic baseline levels.

2. Veins in animals often shift and roll on needle insertion. Stabilizing the vein before venipuncture whenever possible yields better results. Proficiency is gained through experience.

3. Vessel visualization is improved by clipping the fur over the venipuncture site. The skin is then cleansed with an appropriate antiseptic that will not interfere with the study or test being done.

4. Evacuated systems (i.e., Vacutainers) can be used for venipuncture in larger animals. However, in smaller species, a needle and syringe are often used to avoid vessel collapse.

5. Surgical gloves are generally not required unless a transmissible disease is suspected.

6. Use only dry, sterile equipment that is appropriately sized for the species being tested. In general, the gauge and length of the needle are determined by the size and location of the vein being used.

7. As with all venipuncture, the bevel of the needle should be held up and parallel to the vein. Slow, steady aspiration prevents hemolysis and vessel collapse.

8. When repeat samples are required over an extended period, an indwelling **vascular implant** is often better tolerated by the animal. Repeat sampling at too-frequent intervals can lead to resentment.

9. Blood-to-anticoagulant ratios should be monitored, especially when small quantities of blood are used. Results reported from improper ratios can be spurious.

10. Animals should be fasted before sampling to avoid postprandial lipemia.

11. Anesthesia should be employed whenever possible to avoid animal discomfort and to facilitate prompt and simple sampling.

12. After venipuncture, animals should be monitored to ensure that hemostasis is complete.

Phlebotomy is undertaken in animals for many of the same reasons it is performed in humans; however, obtaining the samples requires knowledge of animal anatomy and restraint techniques particular to that species. Table 8–1 provides locations for phlebotomy and the average sample volumes available from the species.

Canine Venipuncture

In the dog, the most common sites for venipuncture are the **jugular,** cephalic, and **recurrent tarsal veins.** Each requires a different restraint technique.

Jugular Vein. The jugular vein in the dog is easily visualized and **tapped** if the fur of the ventral neck is clipped and the dog is in the correct position (Fig. 8–1). An assistant, using the left hand, extends the dog's head and neck and, with the right hand and arm, controls the dog's front legs and feet. The phlebotomist places a thumb in the jugular furrow to distend the vein. The vein is tapped, the sample is collected,

table **8–1** **PHLEBOTOMY LOCATIONS AND AVERAGE SAMPLE VOLUMES, BY SPECIES**

Species (wt)	Location (vein)	Average sample volume (ml)
Dog (20 kg)	Jugular	200
	Cephalic	Variable; 2–10 avg.
	Tarsal	Variable; 2–5 avg.
Cat (3.6–4.5 kg)	Jugular	30
	Cephalic	Variable; 1–2 avg.
	Femoral	Variable; 1–3 avg.
	Marginal ear	Drops
Rabbit (4–6 kg)	Cardiac	50
	Marginal ear	20
	Central ear artery	40–65
Rat (250–400 gm)	Cardiac	2.5
	Jugular	0.3–0.5
	Tail	0.2–0.4
	Retro-orbital plexus	Capillary tube
Mouse (20–40 gm)	Cardiac	0.3
	Tail	Drops
	Retro-orbital plexus	Capillary tube
Guinea pig (750–1000 gm)	Cardiac	5
	Ear	0.1
	Jugular	1
	Medial saphenous	3

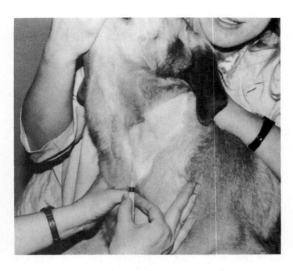

figure **8−1**

Technique for tapping the jugular vein in a dog.

and the needle is withdrawn. The phlebotomist or the assistant then maintains pressure over the site to prevent a hematoma.

Cephalic Vein. The cephalic vein is usually adequate for obtaining blood samples of 2 to 5 ml in large-breed dogs. Clipping the fur of the dorsal foreleg helps in visualizing the vein. An assistant holds the dog on the table and places a restraining arm under the chin and neck; the dog is held close to the assistant's body. The phlebotomist grasps the cephalic vein at the level of the elbow and rolls it outward with thumb pressure. Then, holding the foreleg firmly extended about the area of the

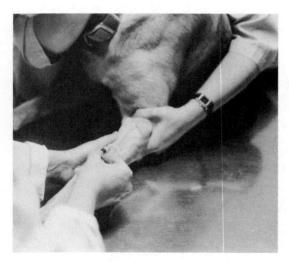

figure **8−2**

Technique for tapping the cephalic vein in a dog.

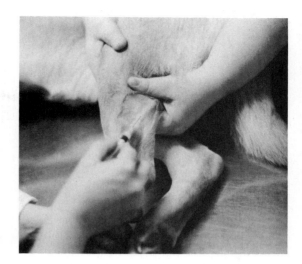

figure **8-3**

Technique for tapping the recurrent tarsal vein in a dog.

wrist, the phlebotomist starts the venipuncture between the wrist and the elbow (Fig. 8-2).

Recurrent Tarsal Vein. Another venipuncture site is the recurrent tarsal vein, which is located on the outside lower hind leg. Because this vein moves easily subcutaneously and is hard to anchor firmly, taking blood from this site can be challenging if the phlebotomist is inexperienced. Once this technique is mastered, however, this site provides the phlebotomist with an excellent alternative to traditional venipuncture locations. It is particularly useful in fractious animals or animals that are head-shy, because it keeps personnel well away from the head (Fig. 8-3).

The dog is placed on its side. The assistant holds the underforeleg and applies pressure to the dog's neck with a forearm to keep the dog's head and neck on the table. The upper rear leg is held firmly above the knee, and the phlebotomist pulls it to extension. This occludes the vessels and provides some stabilization for the venipuncture. Some technicians apply a light tourniquet to further occlude the vessel, although this is seldom needed.

Feline Venipuncture

For cats, venipuncture is best attempted in a quiet environment and at an unhurried pace. Gentle yet firm restraint yields the best result. The most common venipuncture sites in the cat are the jugular, cephalic, and femoral veins; the marginal ear vein can be used in select cases.

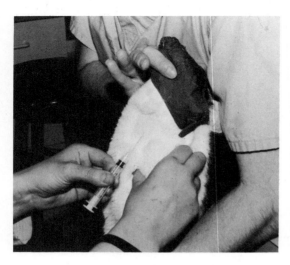

figure **8-4**

Technique for tapping the jugular vein in a cat.

Jugular Vein. The same technique used for the dog can be used in the cat for jugular taps; however, a second technique can be useful in a nervous or fractious animal. The cat's body is snugly wrapped in a heavy towel and placed on its side. The head and neck are left exposed; if necessary, a soft cloth muzzle may also be used. An assistant extends the head and neck with one hand, using the other hand to cradle the towel next to his or her body. The phlebotomist then has a clear view of the jugular vein and can proceed to place a thumb in the jugular furrow and tap the exposed vein (Fig. 8-4).

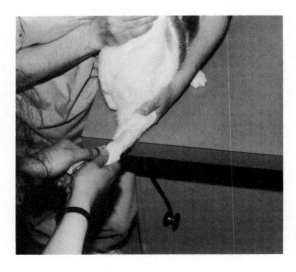

figure **8-5**

Technique for tapping the cephalic vein in a cat.

Cephalic Vein. For a cephalic vein tap in the cat, the same technique used in the dog may be employed, but a few modifications may be of some assistance with a refractory animal (Fig. 8–5). Again, the cat can be snugly wrapped in a heavy towel, exposing only the head and one forelimb. Cats that attempt to bite can be muzzled with a soft cloth muzzle (see Fig. 8–4). Because these muzzles also cover the eyes, they seem to calm the animal greatly.

Femoral Vein. The **femoral vein** in the cat is an underutilized venipuncture site that affords low patient stress and high operator safety. One disadvantage is that the vein moves easily subcutaneously, and hematomas often form at this venipuncture site. However, practice using this site can minimize hematoma formation, and good results can be expected.

The cat is held on its side or rolled snugly in a heavy towel with one hind leg exposed. The fur on the inner thigh is clipped, and an assistant applies digital pressure above the vein. The phlebotomist uses a thumb to stabilize the vein and then completes the venipuncture. Hematoma production is reduced if the assistant places firm pressure over the needle exit site (Fig. 8–6).

Marginal Ear Vein. The marginal ear vein is used only if small amounts of blood are required. The drops obtained are enough to make blood smear slides or to fill a microhematocrit tube.

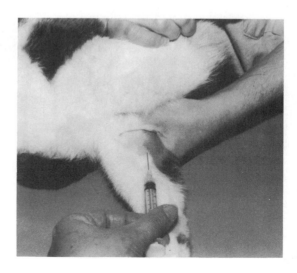

figure **8–6**

Technique for tapping the femoral vein in a cat.

Rabbit Venipuncture

Rabbits are gentle by nature and should be handled in the same way. Many restraining devices are commercially available, but often a large blanket or heavy towel will achieve the same results.

The two most common sites for venipuncture in the rabbit are the heart and the vasculature of the ear. Cardiac puncture requires the use of anesthesia, whereas the ear vessels can be tapped without sedation.

Cardiac Puncture. For cardiac puncture, the anesthetized rabbit is placed in the right lateral recumbent position, and the left chest wall is palpated for the area of maximum heart impulse. An 18- to 21-gauge, 1½ inch needle is used to puncture the heart, and the sample is obtained. Even with a skilled operator this technique can result in pericardial bleeding and trauma to the heart and lungs, and it carries the risk of general anesthesia. In most cases the marginal ear vein is an acceptable and safe alternative.

Marginal Ear Vein. The marginal ear vein of the rabbit is easily located, as it runs along the edge of the ear. The fur over the vessel should be clipped to help visualize the vein (Fig. 8–7). The rabbit is gently but firmly restrained by an assistant, or it can be placed in a restraining box. The vein is occluded and stabilized with pressure from the finger and thumb on each side of the ear base. A drop of xylene to the tip of the ear can be used to further dilate the vessel, if needed. Usually a 20- to 23-gauge, 1-inch needle will yield good results. Although

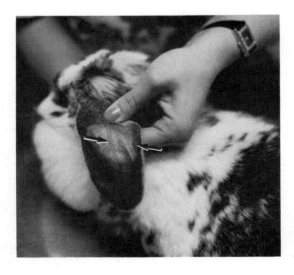

figure **8–7**

Rabbit ear vessels. *Left arrow,* Central ear vessel; *right arrow,* marginal ear vessel.

general anesthesia is not required, a local anesthetic cream (EMLA 5% Cream [lignocaine-prilocaine], Astra Pharmaceutical Ltd., Kings Langley, England) works well to decrease discomfort and may be especially valuable for inexperienced operators.

Rat and Mouse Venipuncture

The most common sites for venipuncture in the rat and mouse include the heart, the tail vein, and the **retro-orbital plexus.** The jugular vein can also be used in the rat. All require general anesthesia.

Cardiac Puncture. Cardiac puncture is most easily achieved by placing the animal on its side and palpating the chest wall for the area of maximum heart impulse (Fig. 8–8). A 25-gauge needle on a 3-ml syringe is advanced perpendicularly into the chest wall. Gentle suction is maintained, and the needle is advanced until blood is received into the syringe. Once the cardiac chamber is entered, it is important not to move the needle. The needle can easily dislodge and cause damage to the heart muscle because of the small size of the chambers.

Jugular Vein. The jugular vein can be tapped in rats, but this is not easy without experience, as the overlying tissue has to be surgically displaced. First, the animal is anesthetized, and the ventral neck is shaved. The skin is incised over the jugular vein parallel to the trachea. In some cases subcutaneous fat must be dissected away to expose the jugular vein. A small-gauge (25-gauge or less) needle is used to tap the vein. Inserting the needle through the belly of the pectoral muscle that overlies part of the vein will help prevent hemorrhage once the needle is removed.

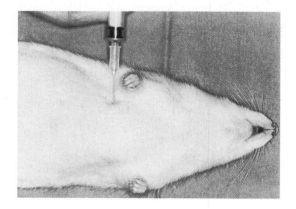

figure **8–8**

Cardiac puncture in a rat. A 20-gauge needle is inserted through the right thoracic wall at the point of maximum heart palpitation. (From Bivin WS: Blood collection and intravenous injection. In Fox JG, Cohen BJ, Loew FM, eds: Laboratory Animal Medicine. New York, Academic Press, 1984, p. 565.)

Tail Vein. The tail vein is the most common vein to be tapped in procedures that the animal is to survive. The lateral tail veins are easily visualized if the tail is warmed before the procedure. This is easily achieved by placing the tail in warm water or under a warming lamp for a few minutes. A small-gauge (25- to 27-gauge) needle is used to enter the tail vein, and gentle suction on the syringe results in collection of a small sample (0.2 to 0.4 ml). A procedure involving snipping the tip of the tail has been described, but this seems unnecessary and I do not advocate it.

Retro-orbital Plexus. Tapping of the retro-orbital plexus is simple to do and provides reliable, albeit small, samples (Fig. 8–9). When executed correctly on an anesthetized animal, it is safe and causes no long-term eye damage. The technique is not without its detractors, however, because of its aesthetically unappealing nature.

A fully anesthetized animal is held on its side with the thumb of the operator occluding the jugular vein just behind the **mandible.** The forefinger of the same hand gently retracts the upper eyelid and produces a slight bulging of the eye. A glass capillary tube is passed into the conjunctiva of the inner canthus of the eye and then is advanced to rupture the orbital sinus. Pasteur pipettes and polyethylene tubing can also be used. The blood flows into the tube by capillary action. When the tube is removed and pressure is released from the jugular vein, blood flow stops promptly. No other form of hemostasis is needed.

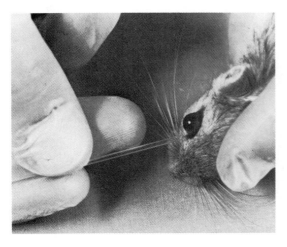

figure **8–9**

Rodent retro-orbital puncture: collection of blood, using a capillary tube, from the orbital sinus of a gerbil. Traction applied by the forefinger produces exophthalmos. (From Bivin WS: Blood collection and intravenous injection. In Fox JG, Cohen BJ, Loew FM, eds: Laboratory Animal Medicine. New York, Academic Press, 1984, p. 565.)

Guinea Pig Venipuncture

Guinea pigs are docile by nature and, if treated as such, are wonderful patients. Because of their gentle nature, quiet disposition, and cleanliness, they are truly easy to keep and make fine laboratory animals. The most common sites for venipuncture in the guinea pig are the heart, ear vein, and jugular vein. The relatively new **medial saphenous** technique also shows promise.

Cardiac Puncture. Cardiac puncture in the guinea pig is similar to that in the rat. The animal is anesthetized and placed on its side. Using a 21- to 23-gauge, 1-inch needle, the heart is entered through the chest wall at the point of maximum cardiac intensity. The smallest gauge needle that will suffice is recommended if the animal is to recover from anesthesia.

Ear Vein. The ear veins in guinea pigs reliably provide small samples of approximately 0.1 ml of blood. As in the rabbit, the ear veins dilate and are more easily visualized if the ear is warmed or a drop of xylene is first applied. Most venipuncture attempts are not made with a needle and syringe because of the small vein diameter. Usually the vein is lanced with a scalpel blade, and the blood is collected in a glass capillary tube or a pipette. Because restraint can be cumbersome, this method is ideally done under anesthesia.

Jugular Vein. The jugular vein is a common venipuncture site, but it requires surgical exposure as described for the rat. Anesthesia and proper surgical technique are required.

Medial Saphenous Vein. The medial saphenous venipuncture site is capable of providing relatively large sample sizes without the risks of cardiac puncture (Fig. 8–10). Sample sizes of up to 3 ml have been consistently obtained.

The animal is anesthetized and placed on its side, and the inner aspect of the hind leg is shaved. The caudal branch of the medial saphenous vein is visible without occlusion of the vessel. A 25-gauge, ⅝-inch needle on a 3-ml syringe is used to enter the vein anywhere along the vessel, although the area between the hock and stifle affords the greatest stability. Digital pressure is applied for 1 minute after exiting the vein to avoid hemorrhage or swelling.

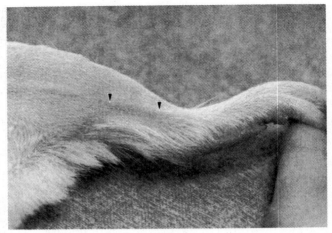

figure **8-10**   Guinea pig saphenous vein is usually readily apparent without manual occlusion after the leg is shaved. The ideal area for venipuncture is outlined by the arrowheads. (From Caraway J, Gray L: Blood collection and intravenous injection in the guinea pig via the medial saphenous vein. Lab Animal Sci 39[6]:623–624, 1989.)

HANDLING BLOOD SAMPLES

Correct technique in obtaining blood samples and proper handling of the blood after it is collected will prevent hemolysis, which is one of the major reasons for incorrect results. Lipemia, the second major reason for spurious laboratory results, is avoided by sampling only fasting animals.

table **8-2**   MECHANISMS BY WHICH HEMOLYSIS AFFECTS LABORATORY RESULTS

Test	Effect	Mechanism
Sodium and chlorine	Decreased	Dilution of constituents in serum
Lactate dehydrogenase, aspartate aminotransferase, alanine aminotransferase, potassium, and phosphorus	Increased	Release of red blood cell constituents into the serum
Plasma protein, fibrinogen	Increased	Increased turbidity
Bilirubin, albumin, calcium, total protein, lipase, creatinine	Variable	Direct color interference

Hemolysis

Hemolysis is the alteration or destruction of red blood cells in such a manner that the hemoglobin is released into the serum/plasma. When the red blood cell membranes are broken and the hemoglobin is liberated, the serum appears pink instead of its normal clear to straw color.

Common causes of hemolysis include the following:

1. Wet equipment
2. Blood samples drawn with too much pressure on the syringe
3. Forcing blood back through the needle and collection syringe into the collection tube
4. Chilled glassware
5. Vigorous mixing of blood with the reagents (gentle inversion is best)
6. Temperature extremes en route to an outside laboratory

Table 8–2 reviews the mechanisms by which hemolysis affects laboratory results.

Lipemia

Lipemia is the presence of an abnormally large amount of lipids in the circulating blood. The amount of lipid circulating is very high after a meal, and if blood is sampled during this period, the resulting serum will be milky white instead of its normal clear yellow color. This increased lipid in the serum will interfere with chemical determinations at the laboratory and give spurious results (Table 8–3). A 12-hour fast before sampling will prevent lipemic serum in most cases. An animal in a diseased state such as hypothyroidism or diabetes mellitus may demonstrate lipemia even after a fast because of the inability of the animal to clear the lipids.

table **8–3**   **EFFECTS OF LIPEMIA**

Test	Effect
Lipase, alanine aminotransferase, aspartate aminotransferase, serum alkaline phosphatase, amylase	Falsely decreased
Total protein, bilirubin, albumin, globulin, calcium, phosphorus, bile acids	Falsely increased

Review Questions

1. A complete blood cell count, white blood cell count, and *Dirofilaria* (heartworm) test are all performed from a _____ tube.
2. A red-top tube provides the laboratory with _____ component of blood that has been centrifuged.
3. The most common sites for venipuncture in the dog are the _____, _____, and _____ veins.
4. The most common sites for venipuncture in the rabbit are the _____ and the _____ veins.
5. Lipemia is best avoided by making sure the animal has fasted for _____ before sampling.

Bibliography

Alleman AR: The effects of hemolysis and lipemia on serum biochemical constituents. Vet Med 85:1272–1284, 1990.

Arrington LR: Introductory Laboratory Animal Science: The Breeding, Care and Management of Experimental Animals. Danville, IL, The Interstate Printers and Publishers, 1972.

Bivin WS, Smith GD: Blood collection and intravenous injection and vascular cannulation. In Fox JG, Cohen BJ, Loew FM, eds: Laboratory Animal Medicine. New York, Academic Press, 1984.

Carraway JF, Gray LD: Blood collection and intravenous injection in the guinea pig via the medial saphenous vein. Lab Anim Sci 39(6):623–624, 1989.

Flecknell PA: Non-surgical experimental procedures. In Tuffery AA, ed: Laboratory Animals: An Introduction for New Experimenters. New York, Wiley-Interscience, 1987, pp. 225–260.

Flecknell PA, Liles JH, Williamson HA: The use of lignocaine-prilocaine local anaesthetic cream for pain-free venipuncture in laboratory animals. Lab Anim 24:142–146, 1990.

Gibbs SR: A simple disposable continuous infusion swivel for unrestrained small animals. J Appl Physiol 70(6):2764–2765, 1991.

Holmes DD: Clinical Laboratory Animal Medicine. Ames, IA, Iowa State University Press, 1984.

Jain NC: Schalm's Veterinary Hematology. 4th ed. Philadelphia, Lea & Febiger, 1986.

Kirk RW, Bistner SI: The Handbook of Veterinary Procedures and Emergency Treatment. 4th ed. Philadelphia, WB Saunders, 1985, pp. 486–496.

MacLeod JN, Shapiro BH: Repetitive blood sampling in unrestrained and unstressed mice using a chronic indwelling right atrial catheter apparatus. Lab Anim Sci 38(5):603–608, 1988.

Miale JB: Laboratory Medicine Hematology. 6th ed. St. Louis, CV Mosby, 1982, pp. 859–932.

Mitruka BM, Rawnsley HM: Clinical Biochemical and Hematological Reference Values in Normal Experimental Animals. New York, Masson Publishing, 1977, pp. 21–39.

Pratt PW: Laboratory Procedures for Animal Health Technicians. Santa Barbara, CA, American Veterinary Publications, 1985.

Sarlis NJ: Chronic blood sampling techniques in stress experiments in the rat—a mini review. Anim Technol 42(1):51–59, 1991.

Smith PA, Prieskorn DM, Knutsen C, Ensminger WD: A method for frequent blood sampling in rabbits. Lab Anim Sci 38(5):623–625, 1988.

Wallace J, Gwynne B, Dodd J, Davidson T: Repeated arteriopuncture in the rabbit: A safe and effective alternative to cardiac puncture. Anim Technol 39(2):119–121, 1988.

Willard MD, Tvedten H, Turnwald GH: Small Animal Clinical Diagnosis by Laboratory Methods. Philadelphia, WB Saunders, 1989.

Wills JE, Thornton S, Gardiner DJ: Optimising the use of rabbits for antiserum production. Anim Technol 38(2):99–120, 1987.

Appendix Tables

Appendix Table A lists the type of test, species, tube type, and amount of sample needed. Appendix Table B reviews anticoagulants and the tube stopper color required for each type of test. Many other less common tests performed in laboratory animals are not included in this section. Specific information about these tests can easily be obtained from a reference laboratory.

appendix table **A**   **COMMON LABORATORY TESTS**

Test	Species	Tube Needed	Sample Needed	Amount
Complete blood cell (CBC) count	All	Lavender	AWB	1 ml
Chemistry screen	All	Red/SS	Serum	2 ml
Blood glucose	All	Gray	AWB	1 ml
Dirofilaria (heart-worm test)	Dog	Lavender	AWB	1 ml
Lyme disease/tick serology	Dog	Red/SS	Serum	1 ml
Feline leukemia	Cat			
ELISA		Lavender	AWB	0.2 ml
IFA		None	Slides	2
Feline immunodeficiency virus	Cat			
ELISA		Lavender	AWB	0.2 ml
Western blot		None	Blood-soaked test paper	
Feline infectious peritonitis	Cat	Red/SS	Serum	1 ml
Packed cell volume (PCV)	All	Glass capillary tube	AWB	1 tube
Endocrine assays	All	Red/SS	Serum	1 ml

AWB = anticoagulated whole blood; ELISA = enzyme-linked immunosorbent assay; IFA = indirect fluorescent antibody test; SS = serum separator tube.

appendix table **B** **TUBE TYPES NEEDED FOR VARIOUS TESTS**

Anticoagulant	Stopper Color	Tests
Ethylenediaminetetra-acetate	Lavender	Complete blood cell (CBC) and white blood cell (WBC) counts, platelet estimation, selected toxicolgy
Potassium oxalate	Gray	Blood glucose
Sodium fluoride heparin	Green	Blood gases, serology, osmotic fragility test
Citrate	Blue	Prothrombin time, partial thromboplastin time, fibrinogen and platelet studies
None	Red	Enzymes, electrolytes, serology, selected immunology, selected toxicology, drug testing, electrophoresis, endocrinology, special chemistries

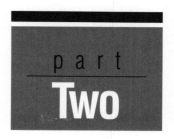

part

TWO

Professional Issues

Interpersonal Communication and Professionalism

John C. Flynn, Jr.

The purpose of this chapter is to discuss the importance of interpersonal communication and professionalism in the day-to-day life of a phlebotomist. The two topics are included in the same chapter because they are intricately related. The chapter concludes with a brief discussion of continuing education, a topic that is very important to all professionals.

EFFECTIVE COMMUNICATION

STAT! The word has different meanings for different individuals in the health care setting. To some it means "drop everything and do it now"; to others it means "do it when I can get to it"; and to still others

135

it may mean something else entirely. STAT is a word that is used every day, but in practice the meaning varies from one individual to another and from one department to another. Therein lies a problem (i.e., effective communication) confronted by phlebotomists.

Communicating is something that laboratory personnel, including phlebotomists, do every day during the course of their jobs. The backgrounds of the people with whom they must communicate are very diversified, as illustrated in Chapter 1 (see Fig. 1–3A, B).

Communication is often thought of as a commodity or substance, as illustrated in the phrase, "we must have more communication"; however, communication is a process, not a thing or an item. For example, if a plant is lacking water, the situation can be corrected by adding more water. However, if there is a "lack of communication," adding more communication does not necessarily correct the problem; in fact, it can make matters worse. In other words, the trouble with communication problems is not always the *quantity* of communication, but instead may be the *quality* of the communication.

A Life Skill

There are certain activities common to all people that can be regarded as life skills. These include maintaining one's health and family relationships, self-evaluation, and decision making. Communication is also a life skill, and yet what training do most people receive in communication? Most have had some grade school and secondary school training in English grammar and composition, and perhaps even some speech training, but generally no interpersonal communications training, which is what phlebotomists, and all laboratory workers, must use daily.

Laboratory workers must realize that there are several levels of communication, all of which must be used properly to do their job well. First is what may be called *intrapersonal* communication. This is the ability to see ourselves as others see us—in another words, "being in someone else's shoes." It also includes the ability to think and plan in advance how to react in a given situation. Second, there is *one-way* communication. An example of this is the sometimes annoying memos or notes received from supervisors, subordinates, or peers. These, if not written properly, are open to improper interpretation. Finally, there is *interpersonal* (two-way) communication, which is the level at which phlebotomists and laboratorians communicate most frequently.

Keys to Successful Communication

Before interpersonal communication can be successful, there are certain fundamental conditions that must be present. First, both parties must be attentive and willing to engage in the communication process. Did you ever try to communicate something to a friend, supervisor, or coworker and at some point notice that they tuned you out? In addition to being a good communicator, the importance of being a good listener cannot be overlooked.

Second, both parties must act as senders and receivers of messages. Once an individual receives a message (by being a good listener) he or she must then become a sender and let the other party know that the message was received and understood, or that more information is needed. The two participants are interdependent; for the communication process to be complete, they must interact.

Finally, and most importantly in the health care setting, communication must be based on mutual understanding. This implies that a given phrase or term, such as "type and hold," means the same thing to both parties. We all have had the experience of being misunderstood because the person we were talking to interpreted something differently from the way we intended. Laboratory personnel must be careful when using **jargon,** which, although used daily in the laboratory, may not be understood outside the laboratory setting.

Obstacles to Successful Communication

Unfortunately, all people encounter barriers to effective communication. One of these is distrust. Distrust can lead to defensive interpersonal communication, especially when the recipient perceives the communication as an attempt to control or manipulate. Additionally, if the sender has a superior attitude, this will trigger a defensive response. Distrust can be overcome if questions or directives are communicated in a nonthreatening way that makes the issue a mutual problem. In this manner, respect and equality are communicated to recipients, giving them the feeling that their help and judgment are valued.

Another common barrier that hinders effective communication is a reference gap. This is analogous to a generation gap or racial gap, in which background and environments affect the way people think, perceive the world or environment, and, in this case, communicate. Phlebotomists have a different frame of reference from others with whom they must communicate, including laboratory personnel in other departments, nurses, physicians, social workers, and patients. For example, you may wonder why a test is ordered STAT. Your frame of reference is different from that of the physician; the physician obviously knows something about the patient that you do not know. Similarly, when you are asked by a physician why a STAT request is not done, you may have to explain that all tests from their service were ordered STAT (an abuse of the

STAT designation) or that an emergency has arisen, thereby communicating to them your frame of reference.

In addition, participants of a health care team often take part in group discussions or decision making. Disagreement with an idea that has been put forth should not be interpreted as personal dislike. This is unhealthy, and it must be realized that all involved in the process have the best intentions, whether the decision is regarding a patient or where to put a new piece of equipment. Furthermore, it should be remembered that in a group process, generally the ultimate decision is usually the best one.

One final issue to be addressed is the use, or often the misuse, of body language. After the spoken word, our eyes are the most potent communicator we possess. Rolling eyes say one thing, and tear-filled eyes, another; surprise, disappointment, and anger are all expressions and feelings we can communicate with our eyes. Reluctance to make eye contact also sends a message to the recipient. Therefore, communication must be both verbal and nonverbal. This is especially important for a phlebotomist, who must interact with patients.

Be sure to make eye contact when speaking or listening to patients. Avoid constant monitoring of the time by either looking at your wristwatch or checking a wall clock. Avoid deep sighs or fidgeting with a pencil, sorting supplies, reading or tapping your toe, all of which signal boredom or impatience. Avoid assuming a defensive posture such as crossing your arms. Your aim is to put the patient at ease, which is best accomplished by acting confident, maintaining eye contact when speaking or listening to a patient or colleague, and appearing relaxed.

Communication Breakdown

For the most part, communication between the phlebotomist and others goes rather smoothly. Communication works well, for example, when a physician or nurse calls for testing results, to determine whether blood is ready for the next day's operation schedule, or to inquire about what color tube is needed for a given test. In these generally relaxed situations, communication is open and friendly. Communication breaks down during times of increased stress, the very times when it is most critical that communication be very smooth. A classic example is when an emergency is occurring either in the emergency department or in the operating room and there is a strain in the communication chain between these places and the laboratory. Someone may ask for results of a test that was never ordered or question why blood is not ready for a trauma victim when the phlebotomist was never informed that there was a trauma victim or that he or she needed to collect a specimen.

General Guidelines for Effective Communication

First, communication should be open and honest. This applies whether you are a **subordinate** or a supervisor, and the key is respect and courtesy for the individual with whom you are communicating. Glibness, deceptiveness, sarcasm, etc., have no place during communication if you wish to be taken seriously.

Second, avoid generalizations and **stereotyping.** We have all been guilty of this at some time, whether it was regarding someone in the health care field or of another race or ethnic group. Talk to the *individual,* for that is what he or she deserves.

Third, consider your "environment" or frame of reference. Explain where you are "coming from," including the pressures and time constraints you are under. It is equally important to consider the environment of the individual with whom you are communicating.

Finally, communicate with a humanistic approach. This implies employing all the above guidelines, in addition to being a good listener.

These guidelines, which are the hallmarks of professional behavior, are summarized in Table 9–1.

In some situations these guidelines cannot be observed. We may be under pressure or short of time, but we must keep in mind that we are dealing with another individual who may not be aware of our circumstances or situation. When the circumstances improve, it is very worthwhile to contact the person with whom we may have been "short" or impatient, explain the situation that led to our abruptness, and thank the person for his or her cooperation and patience. This way we are not forgetting our obligation to a fellow health care provider to be courteous, professional, and, above all else, human.

PROFESSIONALISM

Historically, there were three professions—the law, medicine, and theology (the three "robed" professions)—and three types of professionals—lawyers, doctors, and clergymen. In the nineteenth and

table **9–1**   GENERAL GUIDELINES FOR EFFECTIVE COMMUNICATION

1. Be open and honest.
2. Avoid generalizations.
3. Consider environments.
4. Use a humanistic approach.
5. Be a good listener.

twentieth centuries, the field of professionals greatly expanded to include businesspeople, accountants, computer programmers, social workers, and people in all areas of health care, to name a few.

Strictly speaking, a profession is an area or field that has (1) a distinct field of knowledge requiring specialized training or education; (2) a full-time occupation, often defined and regulated by a peer organization; (3) an occupation that has a service orientation; and (4) a high degree of autonomy. Today, an increasing number of occupations call themselves professions.

Regardless of the definition of a profession, anyone can act professionally while conducting business or employment duties. Professionalism can be thought of as a state of mind. In this sense, acting as a professional encompasses how you look, act, communicate, and present yourself. For a phlebotomist, being well dressed and well groomed is one key to looking like a professional; but looking good is only part of the picture. How you communicate with superiors, peers, and patients and their families is obviously very important to acting professionally. How you conduct yourself and handle adversity will further define whether you act professionally. Obviously, if you throw fits or temper tantrums, act defensively, etc., you are not acting professionally.

One aspect of most professions is the incorporation of a creed or code of ethics into their training. For example, physicians have the Hippocratic oath. However, this oath or creed does not have to be a formal one, but it should include a set of standards to abide by. The American Society for Medical Technology (ASMT) has published a code of ethics that can also be applied to phlebotomists; in summary, this code states that confidentiality will be maintained; duties will be carried out with "accuracy, thoughtfulness and care"; and conduct will always be of a high standard.

Ethical or professional conduct, in general, also includes respect for patients and their rights as outlined in the *Patient's Bill of Rights* (Table 9–2); refraining from discussing patients outside of the proper environment; refraining from anything other than professional communication with patients; and a willingness to assist others.

Finally, one characteristic of a profession is the certification or credentialing of its members. Certification indicates that the individual has mastered the body of knowledge associated with the given profession. Table 9–3 lists the various organizations that offer certification examinations for phlebotomists.

CONTINUING EDUCATION

Once phlebotomists are credentialed and certified, they should not "rest on their laurels." As defined earlier, a profession includes a distinct table **9-2**   **PATIENT'S BILL OF RIGHTS***

1. The patient has the right to considerate and respectful care.
2. The patient has the right to and is encouraged to obtain from physicians and other direct caregivers relevant, current, and understandable information concerning diagnosis, treatment, and prognosis.

   Except in emergencies when the patient lacks decision-making capacity and the need for treatment is urgent, the patient is entitled to the opportunity to discuss and request information related to the specific procedures and/or treatments, the risks involved, the possible length of recuperation, and the medically reasonable alternatives and their accompanying risks and benefits.

   Patients have the right to know the identity of physicians, nurses, and others involved in their care, as well as when those involved are students, residents, or other trainees. The patient also has the right to know the immediate and long-term financial implications of treatment choices, insofar as they are known.
3. The patient has the right to make decisions about the plan of care prior to and during the course of treatment and to refuse a recommended treatment or plan of care to the extent permitted by law and hospital policy and to be informed of the medical consequences of this action. In case of such refusal, the patient is entitled to other appropriate care and services that the hospital provides or transfer to another hospital. The hospital should notify patients of any policy that might affect patient choice within the institution.
4. The patient has the right to have an advance directive (such as a living will, health care proxy, or durable power of attorney for health care) concerning treatment or designating a surrogate decision maker with the expectation that the hospital will honor the intent of that directive to the extent permitted by law and hospital policy.

   Health care institutions must advise patients of their rights under state law and hospital policy to make informed medical choices, ask if the patient has an advance directive, and include that information in patient records. The patient has the right to timely information about hospital policy that may limit its ability to implement fully a legally valid advance directive.
5. The patient has the right to every consideration of privacy. Case discussion, consultation, examination, and treatment should be conducted so as to protect each patient's privacy.
6. The patient has the right to expect that all communications and records pertaining to his/her care will be treated as confidential by the hospital, except in cases such as suspected abuse and public health hazards when reporting is permitted or required by law. The patient has the right to expect that the hospital will emphasize the confidentiality of this information when it releases it to any other parties entitled to review information in these records.
7. The patient has the right to review the records pertaining to his/her medical care and to have the information explained or interpreted as necessary, except when restricted by law.
8. The patient has the right to expect that, within its capacity and policies, a hospital will make reasonable response to the request of a patient for appropriate and medically indicated care and services. The hospital must provide evaluation, service, and/or referral as indicated by the urgency of the case. When medically appropriate and legally permissible, or when a patient has so requested, a patient may be transferred to another facility. The institution to which the patient is to be transferred must first have accepted the patient for transfer. The patient must also have the benefit of complete information and explanation concerning the need for, risks, benefits, and alternatives to such a transfer.

Table continued on following page

table **9-2**   **PATIENT'S BILL OF RIGHTS*** *Continued*

9. The patient has the right to ask and be informed of the existence of business relationships among the hospital, educational institutions, other health care providers, or payers that may influence the patient's treatment and care.
10. The patient has the right to consent to or decline to participate in proposed research studies or human experimentation affecting care and treatment or requiring direct patient involvement, and to have those studies fully explained prior to consent. A patient who declines to participate in research or experimentation is entitled to the most effective care that the hospital can otherwise provide.
11. The patient has the right to expect reasonable continuity of care when appropriate and to be informed by physicians and other caregivers of available and realistic patient care options when hospital care is no longer appropriate.
12. The patient has the right to be informed of hospital policies and practices that relate to patient care, treatment, and responsibilities. The patient has the right to be informed of available resources for resolving disputes, grievances, and conflicts, such as ethics committees, patient representatives, or other mechanisms available in the institution. The patient has the right to be informed of the hospital's charges for services and available payment methods.

The collaborative nature of health care requires that patients, or their families/surrogates, participate in their care. The effectiveness of care and patient satisfaction with the course of treatment depend, in part, on the patient fulfilling certain responsibilities. Patients are responsible for providing information about past illnesses, hospitalizations, medications, and other matters related to health status. To participate effectively in decision making, patients must be encouraged to take responsibility for requesting additional information or clarification about their health status or treatment when they do not fully understand information and instructions. Patients are also responsible for ensuring that the health care institution has a copy of their written advance directive if they have one. Patients are responsible for informing their physicians and other caregivers if they anticipate problems in following prescribed treatment.

Patients should also be aware of the hospital's obligation to be reasonably efficient and equitable in providing care to other patients and the community. The hospital's rules and regulations are designed to help the hospital meet this obligation. Patients and their families are responsible for making reasonable accommodations to the needs of the hospital, other patients, medical staff, and hospital employees. Patients are responsible for providing necessary information for insurance claims and for working with the hospital to make payment arrangements, when necessary.

A person's health depends on much more than health care services. Patients are responsible for recognizing the impact of their life-style on their personal health.

Conclusion

Hospitals have many functions to perform, including the enhancement of health status, health promotion, and the prevention and treatment of injury and disease; the immediate and ongoing care and rehabilitation of patients; the education of health professionals, patients, and the community; and research. All these activities must be conducted with an overriding concern for the values and dignity of patients.

Reprinted with permission of the American Hospital Association, copyright 1992.
* These rights can be exercised on the patient's behalf by a designated surrogate or proxy decision maker if the patient lacks decision-making capacity, is legally incompetent, or is a minor.

table **9-3**   PHLEBOTOMY CERTIFICATION EXAMINATION OPTIONS

American Society of Clinical Pathologists (ASCP)
2100 West Harrison Street
Chicago, IL 60612-3798
(This is probably the most popular examination.)

National Certification Examination
2021 L Street, NW, Suite 400
Washington, DC 20036
(Offered in cooperation with the ASMT.)

American Society of Phlebotomy Technicians (ASPT)
P.O. Box 1831
Hickory, NC 28603

National Phlebotomy Association (NPA)
2623 Bladenburg Road NE
Washington, DC 20018

field of knowledge. Knowledge is not stagnant, and what is regarded as today's truth may be tomorrow's fiction. New theories and methods are being discovered and tested every day on topics ranging from losing weight, to treating patients and illness, and to coping with stress. This is also true in phlebotomy; some examples of changes include the use of evacuated tubes instead of syringes, and keeping the arm straight rather than bent after collecting a blood specimen.

Once you are credentialed and working, how do you learn about new techniques and changes in the field? Some learn from a sales representative, by attending a workshop, or by having an inservice program at their place of employment. This type of learning is known as continuing education (CE).

CE is rapidly growing in importance. Physicians, lawyers, teachers and those in many other professional groups participate in CE and are often required to accumulate CE credits. (Generally, it takes 8 to 10 hours of contact time, depending on the organization, to earn one continuing education unit [CEU].) Once you are certified, some organizations, such as the American Society for Medical Technology and the American Society of Phlebotomy Technicians (see Table 9-3), require accumulation of CEUs to maintain certification. Many other certification and credentialing organizations do not require CE, but they all strongly encourage it. Additionally, the Joint Commission on Accreditation of Healthcare Organizations (JCAHO) requires inservice training.

Most of the above-mentioned organizations provide educational experiences for individuals to earn CEUs, such as workshops at local and national meetings, videoconferences, audioconferences, and self-instructional units. Other noncredentialing organizations, such as the American Association of Blood Banks and the American Association of Clinical Chemistry, offer CE that is recognized by the credentialing organizations. Still other organizations, such as the National Laboratory Training Network and the Area Health Education Center, provide educational opportunities for laboratory personnel. The Mayo Medical Laboratories also offer workshops for phlebotomists at various locations around the country.

As you can see, there is ample opportunity for phlebotomists to acquire CE. As a professional, you should want to continue your education and keep abreast of changes and new technologies in your field. In addition, not only should you attend your organization's CE offerings, but you should also become active in your organization. Volunteer to assist at workshops by organizing and scheduling speakers, rooms, or refreshments. Do not "rest on your laurels." Instead, attend CE (you may not have a choice), and become active in the organization of your choice.

 # Review Questions

1. Activities such as maintaining one's health, self-evaluation, and decision making are examples of _____.
2. The ability to see ourselves as others see us is known as _____ communication.
3. When our background and environment are different from those who we communicate with, this can be referred to as a _____.
4. An occupation with a high degree of autonomy, service orientation, and specialized training is known as a _____.
5. _____ is an activity that is provided by most employers and professional organizations.

Bibliography

Barrack MK: How we communicate; the most vital skill. Macomb, IL, Glenbridge Publishing, 1988.

Duldt BW, Giffin K, Patton BR: Interpersonal Communication in Nursing. Philadelphia, FA Davis, 1984.

Ellis A, Beattie G: The Psychology of Language and Communication. New York, Guilford Press, 1986.

Gazda GM, Childers WC, Walters RP: Interpersonal Communication: A Handbook for Health Professionals. Rockville, MD, Aspen, 1982.

Giffin K, Patton BR: Fundamentals of Interpersonal Communication. 2nd ed. New York, Harper & Row, 1976.

Walton D: Are You Communicating? You Can't Manage Without It. New York, McGraw-Hill, 1989.

Weaver RL: Understanding Interpersonal Communication. 2nd ed. Glenview, IL, Scott, Foresman, 1978.

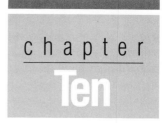
Phlebotomy Unit Management

Dorothy Pfender

The concept of phlebotomy as an individual unit or department is in its infancy. It has only been in recent years that the need for a phlebotomy unit manager has been recognized. The work done in this department is the foundation of the laboratory. The results of tests performed by the best trained technician, on state-of-the-art, properly maintained equipment would be useless to the physician if the specimen were improperly collected or transported. Furthermore, the phlebotomy department acts as a liaison between the laboratory and hospital departments, physicians, patients, and the public. In fact, public opinion of the laboratory is often based on the treatment received in or from the phlebotomy department.

The manager of this department should possess all the managerial skills and training required for the management of any other department.

He or she should be especially capable in relating to people, communicating, organizing, and adapting. The manager of a phlebotomy unit should also have training and skill in phlebotomy techniques. In addition, some understanding of the performance and meaning of the tests for which the specimens are collected is helpful.

ORGANIZATION

Planning

When planning a phlebotomy department, the following should be considered:

1. Number of patients to be served
2. Source of patients (e.g., hospital, physicians' offices, health promotion programs, mass screening, employee physicals)
3. Type of patient (e.g., age, ethnic and religious background, economic status, and whether the patient is in the hospital or ambulatory)
4. Location of the laboratory or laboratories to which specimens will be sent.
5. Type of specimens the department will be collecting (blood, urine, cultures from various sources, blood requiring special pre- or post-treatment, or other bodily excrements)

The information necessary for these considerations can be obtained from the following sources:

1. Hospital administrators
2. Hospital statistics
3. Local or hospital-based physicians
4. Nurses
5. Laboratory directors, managers, and statistics
6. Other skilled health departments (e.g., radiology, respiratory medicine, physical therapy, and nutrition)

Location and Facilities

The location and physical layout of the phlebotomy unit are important. The unit should be easily accessible to **ambulatory** patients from the central registration area and the outside entrance. It should also be located so that phlebotomists have easy access to the emergency department and elevators to patient areas.

The phlebotomy unit should have a reception area that is readily visible to people entering the unit. Requests of ambulatory patients are reviewed here and all necessary patient information obtained and recorded. A computer system (the hospital's or the unit's) is recommended for this work. Ambulatory traffic through the unit is directed from this area. All telephone calls are received here and directed to the proper location.

There should be a paging system or "beepers" available for use by phlebotomists when they are out of the unit area. It is a good idea to have a system by which phlebotomists keep the control desk aware of their location so that they can be informed of new requests received from that area or from an area they will pass on their way back to the laboratory. This increases efficiency and prevents irritation.

Ideally, there should be a phlebotomy information and work organization center. Here requests can be sorted, work organized, and collection notes made. In addition, special instructions and communications can be posted here.

The actual venipuncture area should be private and should contain a comfortable chair for the patient with an area on which to place either arm comfortably. The armrest areas should be at a comfortable height for the phlebotomist; most phlebotomy chairs have adjustable arms. Each area should be equipped with a "panic button" or some other system of requesting help if needed. There should be adequate supplies neatly stored, as well as a sink and biohazard disposal containers in each area. It is advantageous to provide an examination table or a way of allowing the patient to lie down if required. A place should be provided in each area to hang patients' coats; a couple of hooks and a few hangers are usually sufficient. If patients must hang their coats outside the venipuncture area, a secure place should be provided nearby to put patients more at ease.

When each venipuncture area cannot be equipped with a place for the patient to lie down, there must be at least one such area centrally located (1) for patients undergoing a blood test that requires rest before the specimen is collected and (2) for those who experience adverse reactions. Oxygen and ammonia inhalants should be readily available in each room or in the central reclining area. Ideally, all venipuncture areas should be soundproof. This allows private discussions and reactions to the procedures. If children or mentally retarded patients are treated, at least one soundproof room should be available.

Restrooms should be adequate and should be located next to or across the hall from the venipuncture areas. Each restroom should be equipped with some type of emergency call system. Convenient shelf space should be provided for containers and other equipment used before and after collecting the specimen.

It is often advantageous to have the patient collect a urine specimen while waiting for the phlebotomist. The container to be used should be labeled when it is given to the patient. To prevent embarrassment, provide a place where the patient may leave the labeled specimen before returning to the waiting room. This should be convenient to the restrooms and venipuncture areas.

STAFFING

Workload Units

The staffing pattern will differ for each phlebotomy unit. The College of American Pathologists (CAP) and other organizations have published rules for determining how many employee hours are needed and have determined weighted time units called workload units for each test. One unit represents "one minute of technical, clinical, and aide time" needed for a procedure (Table 10–1). These published figures can only be used as guidelines. Because there are so many variables, each unit must evaluate its own situation and determine its own workload units and needs.

To make this determination, the following factors should be considered:

1. Volume of specimens. This is not the number of patients, but the number of tests ordered on each patient. For example, it will take less time to collect blood for a blood glucose test on each of 10 patients than to collect blood for a blood glucose test and a complete blood cell (CBC) count on each of 10 patients.

2. Number and location of patients.

3. Type of patients (i.e., ambulatory patients or inpatients). For inpatients, the time required to reach their room or to go from room to room must be considered. The place of collection (i.e., regular hospital room or special areas) must also be considered. Isolation units or intensive care units, for example, require special preparations to work in them. Even in regular rooms, the problems that the phlebotomist encounters in accessing the patient because of the arrangement of furniture and the

---

table **10–1**   SAMPLE OF CAP WORKLOAD UNITS

Procedure	Workload Units
Capillary puncture on outpatient	8.0
Capillary puncture on inpatient	14.0
Venipuncture on outpatient	4.0
Venipuncture on inpatient	10.0

presence of visitors should be considered. Children, elderly patients, and burned or trauma patients may also require more time.

4. Method of labeling specimens (preprinted labels or hand written).

5. The amount of work that can be done at scheduled collection times.

6. The number of STAT or special collections that are required.

7. The size of the emergency department, trauma unit, and other specific patient units. In some hospitals, one or all of these units may be large enough to support an assigned phlebotomist or person to handle the transportation of specimens.

8. Whether the department offers 24-hour coverage or has another department cover evening and night hours.

9. Duties other than collecting specimens (i.e., logging in specimens, centrifuging specimens, and preparing specimens to be mailed or picked up).

Experience has proven that it is most efficient to have a core of full-time employees to cover the basic needs and a staff of part-time employees for peak hours and other times of staff shortages. The manager should try to schedule enough phlebotomists so that they do not feel constantly pushed, but not so many that they are bored. Be realistic when allotting time required to collect specimens.

Training and Professional Attributes

Employ formally trained phlebotomists if possible, and develop an orientation and instruction program for these employees; generally 2 weeks is sufficient. This program should be longer, if necessary, to familiarize the employee with the methods, procedures, and general operating protocol of the department. A department manual should be provided, and employees should understand that uniformity is necessary. Physicians compare results of tests done before and after treatment, and uniformity of test performance is necessary for these comparisons to be valid. If you employ less experienced phlebotomists, the orientation and training period must be longer and more in depth.

In addition to formal education and training, phlebotomists should possess the following professional attributes:

1. Professional appearance

2. Ability to relate well to people by showing concern and being courteous

3. Ability to remain calm during emergencies

4. Capacity to accept changes

5. Willingness to adhere to the rules of the department

6. Capacity to admit and correct problems

OPERATIONAL PLAN

It is important to develop goals and objectives for the department. The hospital or clinic will probably have general goals with which you will be expected to identify. However, more specific goals are needed to develop an efficient, successful department. The primary goal of every phlebotomy department is to contribute to good patient care by obtaining proper (good) specimens for the tests requested by the physician. This means that specimens must be collected from the proper patient, at the correct time, using the proper technique; all specimens must be labeled correctly and transported in a timely manner to the testing department.

A well-organized system of handling requests and a collection routine for these specimens is required to accomplish this goal. A smoothly functioning work plan is difficult to develop. It requires a lot of thought and planning with many other departments involved in the care of patients. The phlebotomy department shares servicing the patient with radiology, respiratory therapy, physical therapy, nursing, and dietary staffs; physicians; and possibly others. It is important that all staff members feel that they are part of a team and work as such. This necessitates that each department understand and respect the work requirements of the others. Regular meetings with managers or representatives from all departments are recommended. The requirements of the procedures in each department should be discussed. When there are conflicts, reasons why changes can or cannot be made should be presented. Departments must work together to reach solutions that allow each department to organize its work satisfactorily. Usually, the phlebotomy department must take the initiative in this team effort, as it is the department most affected by the work of all other departments. If you are honest about your needs and try to be flexible, others will usually follow your example, and in this way a mutually satisfactory work organization can be developed.

Explain to your employees the reasons for any compromises either by your department or by others. This will develop a good rapport among all departments. This approach helps to create an understanding and respect for the employees and needs of all departments, yours included.

COLLECTION SCHEDULE

A specified time for early morning specimen collection (i.e., morning rounds) is a given in all hospitals. At this time routine, fasting, and presurgical specimens are collected. The time of collection and the number of employees involved varies, depending on the following:

1. When the laboratory wants the specimen. If the laboratory day shift starts at 7 A.M. and these technicians set up the instruments, they will not be ready for the specimens until sometime after 7 A.M. If the night technicians set up the instruments and the day shift starts at 7 A.M., the laboratory will be ready for specimens at 7 A.M.

2. Who is responsible for recording and preparing specimens for analysis. If a department other than the analyzing department does this, it will need the specimens at a time that will allow it to meet the laboratory starting time.

3. Volume of specimens, including the number (how many tubes) and type (do they require special handling?).

4. Number and location of patients. Are they in rooms that are close to each other? Are they in special areas that require special preparation?

5. Type of patient (e.g., children, elderly patients, or burn patients).

6. When breakfast is served.

The morning collection usually starts between 5:30 and 7:00 A.M.

Several other collection times scheduled throughout the day will help with the organization of the work. Three other scheduled collection times are recommended: mid-morning, mid-afternoon, and early evening. The times you choose for your scheduled rounds will vary with your needs. Times that have proven satisfactory are 11:00 A.M., 2:30 P.M., and 7:00 P.M. All requests received in the laboratory up to 15 minutes before a scheduled collection should be included in that collection. If the departments involved understand what is done at these scheduled times, many telephone calls and false STAT requests can be eliminated.

STAT and other special collection requests are a big part of every day's work. It is impossible to predict how many and when these requests will be received. It seems logical to have them handled by whoever is not busy at the time the requests are received, which works well unless everyone or no one is busy. When no one is busy, some people never volunteer. When everyone is busy, there is controversy over who should interrupt what they are doing. Thus, it is necessary to have a schedule assigning STAT collection as a primary responsibility for designated periods of time. Two-hour periods work well, especially if the laboratory receives several STAT requests. The STAT phlebotomist should be expected to be involved in the routine work when possible. It is important to have a written procedure to be followed when a phlebotomist receives a STAT request while engaged in routine work. Establish a routine to be used by the STAT phlebotomist to transfer routine work to a previously determined phlebotomist. This will eliminate the need to make decisions under stress. Make the STAT assignments as equitably as possible. Honor requests for assignments, but check regularly to be sure that assignments are satisfactory to the entire staff and you.

Establish methods and procedures carefully. It is wise to obtain input from all concerned before making your decision and to share the basis of your decision with all persons involved. When your choice is made, insist on uniformity. In some instances (e.g., Ivy bleeding time tests), uniformity is essential for results to be useful to the physician. In other circumstances, minor personal variations may be accepted. This should be kept to a minimum and should not be allowed if the variation could affect the results. The more uniform the department's techniques, the better its performance can be evaluated.

Occasionally, reorganization will be necessary to accommodate changes in the hospital, laboratory, or department. Have all other departments review the proposed changes for possible conflicts. If any conflicts arise, resolve them before instituting the change. Provide all departments with the necessary facts of the change and when it will become effective, and distribute this information in writing.

EQUIPMENT MANAGEMENT

The equipment, both expendable and **capital,** used in the phlebotomy department should be chosen carefully. The decision regarding what to obtain should be made in cooperation with the phlebotomists and in line with budget considerations.

Expendable Equipment

Expendables should be chosen carefully after the unit manager and the phlebotomists have used them and discussed their advantages and disadvantages. Do not buy based on price alone, and choose only one kind. Uniformity of equipment is economical, space saving, and important to the operation of the department. Stock the variety of sizes that you need from the same manufacturer whenever possible. See Table 10–2 for a list of expendables.

Storage space is almost always a problem. All products are dated, and you should have approximately 2 months' supply on hand. Determine from statistics and operating experience what your yearly need will be. When you place an order for a year's supply, you are assured that the product will be there for you. Generally, you will also receive bulk and guaranteed pricing for the year. Make an agreement with your supplier to deliver your order in designated portions at designated intervals. A good plan is to have one-thirteenth of your yearly order delivered at a given date, another delivery 2 weeks later, and remaining deliveries every 4 weeks afterward.

---

table **10-2**   EXAMPLES OF EXPENDABLE EQUIPMENT

Needles	Adhesive bandages
Syringes	Glass slides
Lancets	Gloves
Tubes	Biohazard/sharps containers
Tourniquets	Labeling pens
Alcohol, alcohol pads	Special labels/precautions
Povidone-iodine swabs	Puncture site warmers
Cotton balls	Ammonia inhalants
Gauze, sterile pads	Clay sealer
Adhesive tape	

Expendable supplies used in small quantities should be ordered at intervals, with quantities determined by usage, storage space, and order processing and delivery time. It is wise to keep at least 2 weeks' supply in stock.

Capital Equipment

Collection trays are a vital piece of capital equipment; each phlebotomist should have his or her own. The organizing and stocking of the tray is very personal, and phlebotomists prefer not to share trays. The collection volume and the space in which they are used and stored must be considered when selecting size and shape. The construction and weight of the tray is also an important consideration.

Capital equipment should be evaluated carefully. Consider the following:

1. How well it meets your needs
2. Accuracy
3. Reproducibility
4. Ease of operation
5. Ease of maintenance
6. Available service
7. Whether quality control is available

It is important to see the equipment demonstrated and, when possible, to obtain opinions from other users. See Table 10-3 for a list of capital equipment that may be needed for a phlebotomy unit.

table **10-3**   EXAMPLES OF CAPITAL EQUIPMENT

Collection trays
Venipuncture chairs
Beds or other reclining surfaces
Utility carts and cabinets
Refrigerators
File cabinets
Computer
Blood pressure cuffs
Racks for tubes
Glucose screening instruments
Hemoglobuin and/or hematocrit screening instruments
Beepers and/or communication system
Alarm systems
Timers
Stopwatches
Centrifuges

Inventory

Maintain an **inventory** of all supplies and equipment. A biweekly inventory of expendables will serve to alert you to unexpected shortages and excesses. This allows time to order or change prescheduled deliveries. Capital equipment should be labeled and records kept of its location, use, and maintenance.

MAINTAINING QUALITY

Safety, quality control, and quality assurance programs should be developed to maintain quality. Guidelines for these programs are supplied by the Joint Commission on Accreditation of Healthcare Organizations (JCAHO), the College of American Pathologists (CAP), and the Occupational Safety and Health Administration (OSHA).

Record Keeping

Records should be kept of preventive maintenance, repairs, and controls run on all equipment. Temperature of refrigerators and water baths should be recorded daily. Regular review of these records will help maintain the quality of the department's work. Accrediting agencies and the federal government have established mandatory periods of time for which all records must be kept available. This varies, but 5 years is the most common requirement.

Practical and useful systems for monitoring the safety, quality control, and quality assurance programs of the department should be established. Such monitoring can point out weak areas in planning, organizing, budgeting, etc., as well as the progress and successes of the department. The value of these records should be explained to the staff. Review these records regularly, and share your opinion of their meaning with the members of the department. Be sure to commend staff members when results are good, and thoroughly discuss any indicated improvement when results are less than acceptable.

Continuing Education

As discussed in Chapter 9, a system of continuing education should also be developed and implemented. Make available to employees information about advances in the areas of health care in which they are involved. Encourage them also to become familiar with developments in other areas of health care. Encourage attendance at seminars and workshops by providing financial aid and an equitable distribution of opportunity. Be sure you, as a manager, attend seminars and workshops and keep informed of advances in the field.

Communication

When other department managers meet to discuss new techniques or problems, take a representative from your department with you. Your staff members are frequently more aware of conflicts with their work than you are. Including them also strengthens the team effort concept.

Have formal, documented inservice programs for all changes in techniques, supplies, or work routines. Encourage questions and discussion to prevent misunderstandings. Regular department meetings should be conducted to share any information about the department or things that might affect the department. Encourage employees to share any information, problems, or concerns they might have about the department. In this way you can "iron out" wrinkles and attempt to create a closely knit department.

Employee Performance and Review

Develop job descriptions and, when possible, create position levels. The levels may be based on responsibilities, education, kind of work, etc. This provides incentive for employees and supplies management with a basis for recognizing exceptional employee performance.

Keep complete and accurate records of the performance of each employee and discuss all entries with him or her. Performances that meet or exceed expectations should be commended and encouragement given. The reason for a less-than-satisfactory performance should be clarified and help offered to correct the problem. These records should be maintained for the duration of employment and retained for the periods dictated by law. Usually the personnel department will have printed guidelines.

BUDGETING

Budgeting, which is a part of every manager's responsibility, is a way of putting a dollar value on your plans. Anticipated revenues and expenditures are determined by considering the following:

1. Volume of work
2. Hours of work
3. Materials
4. Equipment
5. Historical records
6. Future plans
7. Outside services

The two most common systems of budgeting are "grass-roots budgeting" and "zero base budgeting." The system used is usually dictated by the hospital or clinic. Most books on management discuss budgeting in detail (see Bibliography).

SUMMARY

The preceding discussion pertains to phlebotomy units that are part of a hospital or clinic; the details will vary depending on the size and type of institution. A phlebotomy unit that is not part of a hospital or clinic will require the same basic management, although there will be fewer departments with which to coordinate your work. Usually there will be less variety of specimens collected and fewer STAT requests. It will also be necessary to arrange to have a physician available and to have a plan to care for patients who become ill or have adverse reactions. Otherwise, the rules and requirements remain the same.

Review Questions

1. True or false: The public's opinion of the clinical laboratory is often based on their treatment by the phlebotomy department.
2. How may a computer system be used in phlebotomy units?
3. For what type of patient is a soundproof room recommended for phlebotomy?
4. To determine the amount of time needed to complete a test or procedure, managers use _____.
5. Each phlebotomy department should have well-developed _____ and _____.

Bibliography

Becan-McBride K: Textbook of Clinical Laboratory Supervision. New York, Appleton-Century-Crofts, 1982.

College of American Pathologists: Laboratory Workload Recording Methods. Skokie, IL, College of American Pathologists, 1980.

College of American Pathologists: So You're Going to Collect a Blood Specimen — An Introduction to Phlebotomy. 3rd ed. Danville, IL, College of American Pathologists, 1986.

National Committee for Clinical Laboratory Standards: NCCLS Approved Standard: ASH-3 Standard Procedures for the Collection of Diagnostic Blood Specimens by Venipuncture. Villanova, PA, NCCLS, 1991.

Snyder JR, Senhauser DA: Administration and Supervision in Laboratory Medicine. 2nd ed. Philadelphia, JB Lippincott, 1989.

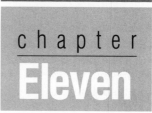
Quality Assurance

Mary E. Paranto

Surviving in today's consumer-oriented market has prompted many organizations to include as part of their mission statement the word "quality": quality products, quality services, quality staff, quality materials. These organizations are committed to quality, as evidenced by the frequently used slogan "customer satisfaction guaranteed." A significant amount of time and resources are spent on ensuring and improving quality, but the benefits — employee satisfaction, improved production, improved teamwork, improved operations, increased market share, increased sales, increased profitability, and respect — become vital to an organization's success.

The health care industry, wanting to retain a competitive advantage in business, has adopted the practice of ensuring quality. Furthermore, as the 21st century approaches, the health care industry will be shifting its focus from quality assurance to continuous quality improvement.[1] Leaders in the health care industry have also included in their mission statements the word "quality." Commitment to, enthusiasm about, and concern for quality patient care equate with success.

The purpose of this chapter is to heighten awareness about quality, to present the general practices of quality assurance, and to apply them to phlebotomy.

QUALITY: DEFINITION AND PRINCIPLES

What is quality? To strive for quality, it is important to know what it is. **Quality** is best defined as a degree of excellence. This definition tends to be most applicable not only to businesses, but also to society-wide issues.

The principles of quality in business lie in fact and perception. Doing the right thing, doing it the right way, doing it right the first time, and doing it on time all are aspects of quality.[2] These aspects of quality, when applied to the health care setting, are often driven by outside agencies, both government (e.g., the Food and Drug Administration [FDA]) and voluntary accrediting agencies (e.g., Joint Commission on the Accreditation of Healthcare Organizations [JCAHO]).

The perceptions of quality include delivering the right product, satisfying the customer's needs, meeting the customer's expectations, and treating every customer with integrity, courtesy, and respect.[2] Even if the aspects of quality are met, will they alone be enough to attract and retain customers?

Achieving balance between the aspects and the perceptions of quality requires constant adjusting. Xerox, Federal Express, and Motorola, Inc., are examples of quality award-winning companies. These and others serve as role models for many health care–oriented businesses.

Quality Assurance vs. Quality Control

Clinical laboratory scientists performed quality work and provided quality results long before the term "quality assurance" became popular. How? By performing quality control. **Quality control** (QC) is the process that validates final results and quantifies variations. When a test (e.g., glucose) is performed on a patient specimen, control samples representing high, low, and normal results are also tested. Decisions about the reportability of the patient's results are made based on a comparison with the results of the control testing. Quality control enables laboratory scientists to confidently report accurate and reproducible test results.

If clinical laboratory practitioners have a close association with quality already, why the increased attention to ensuring it? In addition to economic survival, the pressures of external forces such as accrediting agencies, government regulations, and the public have increased. "Every health-care delivery system has as its major goal the provision of high-quality, cost-effective patient care."[3] **Quality assurance** (QA), to the health care practitioner, is the process of making sure that standards of care have been maintained. The use of laboratory tests to diagnose disease and monitor treatments has significantly increased over time, resulting in a proportionate increase in the importance of ensuring overall laboratory quality. QA takes on a more global view, unlike QC, which is specific (i.e., test or product related). Assuring quality in the laboratory means assessing the entire department's operation to identify areas with negative outcomes and those with positive outcomes (e.g., staff, procedures, training, QC, equipment, computers, and materials/supplies). QC then becomes one part of a QA program. It is possible to have a QC program without having a QA program; this is how laboratories operated for many years. However, it is not possible to have a QA program without a QC program.

BASIC QUALITY ASSURANCE PRACTICES

Participation in a QA program has become part of the laboratory accreditation standards put forth by such groups as the College of American Pathologists (CAP)[4] and the American Association of Blood Banks (AABB).[5] In the health care industry, the JCAHO has been instrumental in providing direction to facilities desiring to implement QA programs. First, it has characterized quality care to be effective, acceptable to the patient, accessible, efficient/appropriate, and continuous/consistent.[6] Second, the JCAHO has outlined 10 steps to take when designing and implementing a QA program (Table 11-1).[7] These include assigning responsibility, identifying important aspects of care, establishing **indica-**

---

table **11-1**   THE JCAHO's 10 STEPS TO A QA PLAN

1. Assign responsibility
2. Delineate scope of care
3. Identify important aspects of care
4. Identify indicators related to these aspects of care
5. Establish thresholds for evaluation
6. Gather and organize data
7. Evaluate care when thresholds are reached
8. Take corrective action
9. Assess the effectiveness of the actions; document improvement
10. Communicate relevant information

tors (i.e., specific, measurable variables) and **thresholds** (i.e., points/ values prompting study of an aspect of care), collecting and analyzing data, taking **corrective action** when indicated (i.e., implementing activities geared toward correcting the problem/situation), monitoring the effectiveness of the corrective action, and reporting this information to the appropriate personnel.

To provide further direction, the JCAHO says a QA program can be designed by focusing attention on the important aspects of care that are high volume, high risk, high cost, or problematic. Involving the health care staff in the entire QA process, from design to evaluation, is also recommended.[7]

A well-directed QA program will enable one to see the components of an operation that need to be corrected to meet and adhere to the standards of care. Just as important, a well-directed program will enable one to see the components of an operation that are already high in quality and cost effective (i.e., not requiring corrective action). Many times the need to improve an aspect of care for one section of a health care facility requires interdepartmental involvement and teamwork. An anticipated benefit from this type of activity is significant improvement in the quality of care delivered by that facility.

The following QA tools can be found in a facility that has quality care as its focus:

1. Information important to decision making is communicated (usually by memorandum, newsletter, staff meetings, or logbook).

2. Orientation and training are well structured (not too long, not too short, and with checklists pertaining to the important aspects of the job).

3. Continuing education is strongly encouraged and, ideally, provided.

4. Performance is monitored by supervisory personnel and compared with standards (not with the performance of coworkers), and an annual appraisal is conducted.

5. Standard operating procedure (SOP) manuals are up-to-date, written by supervisory personnel and citing accrediting and governing agencies' regulations when necessary, reviewed by the director annually, and serve as a reference for all employees.

6. Each employee has a personnel file on record containing items of no surprise to the employee (e.g., job description, performance evaluations, counseling documentation, letters of commendation, etc.).

7. Proficiency/competency tests are distributed to the staff on a rotational basis or given to all staff when sufficient quantity exists to do so.

8. Individual participation in scheduled QC and QA activities are included in the job description.

9. Equipment and instrumentation are calibrated, maintained, and serviced as scheduled.

10. Computer systems are validated before using and monitored thereafter.

11. The workplace and environment is safe.

12. There are leaders who actively seek suggestions.

13. Documentation of all of these items is expected (Table 11–2).

Additional information about these items can be found in Chapters 9 and 10.

PHLEBOTOMY QUALITY ASSURANCE

Aspects of Quality

Performing the right type of phlebotomy (venipuncture vs. skin puncture), doing it the right way (i.e., per procedure), doing it correctly the first time, and doing it on time are the aspects of quality in phlebotomy. Many of these aspects have already been detailed elsewhere in this textbook. Adhering to these procedures is one step toward quality patient care.

The importance of assuring quality in phlebotomy is best stated this way: "A test result is no better than the quality of the specimen received in the laboratory."[8] Having quality technicians/technologists, quality procedures, and quality instrumentation means little if the specimen received in the laboratory is of poor quality. Specimens of low quality can produce inaccurate and potentially dangerous results. This may have a negative and possibly expensive outcome on patient care: the wrong

---

table **11–2**   **TOOLS FOR ASSURING QUALITY**

1. Active two-way communication
2. Well-structured orientation and training
3. Periodic continuing education
4. Monitored and appraised performance
5. Standard operating procedure manuals
6. Accurate personnel file
7. Periodic proficiency/competency testing
8. Participation in QC and QA activities
9. Properly functioning and maintained equipment and supplies
10. Validated and monitored computer systems
11. Safe work environment
12. Leaders who seek suggestions
13. Documentation

treatment may be administered, the wrong patient may be treated, the wrong dosage may be given, the wrong blood type may be transfused, and patient death may even occur as a consequence of an improperly collected specimen. Obviously both the patient and the health care facility want to avoid these situations. Phlebotomists should want to strive for quality in their work so that these negative outcomes can be avoided.

Because blood and other body fluids begin to change immediately after collection from the body, the specimen collector should be trained to take steps that will minimize these changes. These steps include the following:

1. Using and referring to clearly written procedures
2. Using properly designed requisitions and report forms appropriately
3. Using the correct collection technique
4. Transporting the specimen to the laboratory according to procedure.

The laboratory that performs the tests is responsible for preparing the procedure manuals and other important information regarding procurement of blood or body fluid specimens. This information should be provided to every health care professional involved in the phlebotomy process. Adherence to these steps ensures that the specimen, and ultimately the test result, will be an accurate reflection of the patient's condition and lead to a positive patient outcome.

THE PROCEDURE MANUAL FOR SPECIMEN COLLECTION

The most important step in ensuring quality phlebotomy is using and referring to the procedures that describe, outline, and detail specimen collection. Table 11–3 summarizes the contents of specimen collection manuals useful in ensuring quality blood specimens.

Professionals are not expected to remember all of the details in the procedure manual. However, they should know the general content and remember that the manual exists for their reference. It contains answers for most specimen-related questions and should be used when the patient's life is not in jeopardy.

It is my experience that most phlebotomy errors occur because standard operating procedures are not followed. After the training period, when a question comes to mind, the specimen collection manual should be consulted for the answer. In the hospital setting, all nursing units should have a specimen collection manual, as nurses, medical students, and physicians sometimes procure specimens. Therefore, the manual should be accessible to them, as well as to the phlebotomist, at all times. The laboratory supervisor should be contacted when the procedure is unclear, thought to be outdated, or difficult to find.

table **11-3**	SPECIMEN COLLECTION MANUAL: CONTENTS USEFUL IN ASSURING QUALITY SPECIMENS

1. The following should be included for each test:
   a. Test name and alternative name(s)
   b. Patient preparation
   c. Type of specimen
   d. Timing requirements
   e. Type of tube/container
   f. Transportation requirements
   g. Labeling requirements
   h. Test requisition form or code
   i. Name and telephone number of laboratory
2. Criteria for unacceptable specimens
3. Steps for handling inability to collect specimen
4. Requirements for acceptable newborn/pediatric samples

Each test performed in the laboratory is addressed in the specimen collection manual. The test name, including alternative names, notes on how to prepare the patient for the test (e.g., fasting), the type of preferred specimen (e.g., venous), notes on timing requirements (e.g., for glucose tolerance tests), and the type of container in which to collect the specimen (e.g., ethylenediaminetetra-acetate Vacutainer tube) should be included. Transportation requirements emphasizing the effects of time, temperature, exposure to light, and excessive vibration or rough handling can be found in this manual. Adherence to these requirements is critical to certain tests (e.g., bilirubin). Adherence to specimen labeling requirements is also critical for some tests, especially those performed by the blood bank; therefore, labeling procedures are included in the manual.[7] Figure 11-1, a sample page from an existing manual, illustrates many of these items.

The appropriate test requisition form and the name of the laboratory performing the test can be found in the manual, along with the laboratory's telephone number.[7] Interestingly, the test requisition form may be another, more practical source of specimen collection information. As shown in Figure 11-2, many of the items found in the collection manual are also found on the test requisition form.

Unacceptable Specimens. Some specimen collection manuals also include, for each test, the criteria for an unacceptable specimen. Specimen rejection may occur, for example, when (1) labeling is inadequate or improper; (2) collection is not timely (e.g., within a certain number of hours after treatment); (3) the sample volume is insufficient for the test being ordered, especially when the specimen container includes an additive; (4) the wrong collection tube or container is used; (5) a collection tube is used after its expiration date; (6) the sample is transported

TEST	SPECIMEN INSTRUCTIONS	HP*	REFERENCE RANGE	LAB CODE	FEE
BETA-SUBUNIT PREGNANCY TESTS - See HCG listings.					
BETA-2 MICRO-GLOBULIN, SERUM	3 mL blood, red top tube.		20-39 yr: 0-2.0 mg/L 40-59 yr: 0-2.6 60-79 yr: 0-3.1	B2M	40.00
BETA-2 MICRO-GLOBULIN, URINE	Urine 5 mL. Patient must void, then drink large glass of water. Collect urine 1 hour later.		0-250 mcg/L	B2U	40.00
BILE PIGMENT, URINE	25 mL urine, random specimen.		None Detected	UBP	8.00
BILIARY DRAINAGE	Physician must schedule with lab (955-6362 or 6363). Rush specimen to lab in sterile container.			BLD	124.00
BILIRUBIN, TOTAL AND DIRECT	3 mL blood, red top tube.		Total: 0.2-1.2 mg/dL Direct: 0.0-0.4	BIL	23.00
BILIRUBIN, TOTAL MICRO (NEONATAL BILIRUBIN)	Blood; 1 Microtainer. Protect from light.			MBL	50.00
BLASTOMYCOSES	5 mL blood, red top tube. Consultation with lab suggested (955-6363). Fill out microbiology request and case history form.			BLY	13.00

NOTE: Antibody to blastomyces may be significant when interpreted in light of a suggestive clinical picture. CF titers of 1:8 are also suggestive. Higher titers or rising titers are more significant.

TEST	SPECIMEN INSTRUCTIONS	HP*	REFERENCE RANGE	LAB CODE	FEE
BLEEDING TIME (TEMPLATE)	Performed Monday-Friday on day shift. Schedule with lab 1 day in advance (955-7687).		2-8 Minutes	BT	50.00

*HP: Highest lab priority available (S=Stat, A=ASAP)

figure 11-1   Sample page from a laboratory specimen collection manual. (From Laboratory Information Handbook. Philadelphia, Thomas Jefferson University Hospital Clinical Laboratories, September, 1991, p. 24.)

incorrectly (e.g., not sent on ice); and (7) the specimen is found to be hemolyzed (which can adversely affect tests such as potassium). When a specimen is deemed to be unacceptable, it usually must be recollected. Unacceptable specimens, recollected specimens, and duplicate specimen collections are central to the phlebotomy QA process.

Unsuccessful Collection Attempts. In addition to unacceptable specimen criteria, the specimen collection manual should include a procedure listing the steps the phlebotomist can take when unable to collect a blood specimen. This procedure should address unsuccessful venipunctures, patient unavailability, and patient refusal to be tested. In each scenario, documentation (see Figure 11–3) is important for quality review, as the problem must be identified and corrected. Therefore, the number of collection attempts is included as an indicator in the phlebotomy QA program.

Newborn and Pediatric Patients. Finally, the unique handling of newborn and pediatric patients should be covered in the specimen collection procedure manual. Specifically, the minimum amount of blood needed to perform a laboratory test on one of these patients should be highlighted in the manual. An example of pediatric specimen requirements is shown in Figure 11–4. Many premature infants undergo transfusion merely to replace blood removed for laboratory testing (known as iatrogenic blood loss). By collecting the smallest amount of blood required for testing, significant blood loss can be avoided. Because of the small blood volumes in newborns and children, the number of times blood is collected and the amounts removed from these patients should be monitored and included in the phlebotomy QA program.

QUALITY CONTROL OF SUPPLIES AND INSTRUMENTS

One of the best QA practices in phlebotomy resides in the persons trained to perform blood collection procedures. Reports from phlebotomists that evacuated tubes are not working properly (e.g., not drawing the appropriate amount) may result in the performance of a blood collection QC procedure. The implementation of a new brand of tube or of a modified evacuated tube may also be reason to perform a QC procedure.

Blood collection QC procedures may or may not be included in a phlebotomy QA program, depending on the particular facility's interests and experiences. If difficulties are encountered by the workers who use the vacuum tubes, or if new technologies are implemented, the supplier or manufacturer may be contacted and asked to assist with corrective action or provide consultation.

THOMAS JEFFERSON UNIVERSITY HOSPITAL
CLINICAL LABORATORIES

DIRECTOR, REX B. CONN, M.D.

INPATIENT ONLY

☐ **EMERGENCY** ➤ (PHONE NUMBER:
PHONE RESULTS TO
NOTE: STAT SPECIMENS MUST BE BROUGHT DIRECTLY TO LAB OR LAB FLOOR PAVILION, OR SENT VIA THE PNEUMATIC TUBE

| SPECIMEN COLLECTED (REQUIRED BY STATE LAW) | DATE | TIME | ☐ AM ☐ PM |

NAME OF COLLECTOR:

DIAGNOSIS:

(MEDICATION KNOWN OR SUSPECTED)

ISOLATION PRECAUTIONS ☐ YES ☐ NO

SPECIMEN CONTAINER MUST SHOW PATIENT'S NAME

//// STAT //// STAT //// STAT //// STAT //// STAT //// STAT ////

FOR URGENTLY NEEDED RESULTS, CALL LAB BEFORE SPECIMEN IS SENT AND ADVISE RESIDENT OR SUPERVISOR.
TELEPHONE NUMBERS ARE LISTED WITH EACH LABORATORY HEADING.

CODE	TEST	SPECIMEN	RESULT	CODE	TEST	SPECIMEN	RESULT	CODE	TEST	SPECIMEN
	CHEMISTRY X6801				**URINALYSIS X6823**				**TOXICOLOGY X8529**	
☐ SM7	CHEM-7 PANEL	G4	2,3	☐ UA	URINALYSIS	UR		☐ DSE	DRUG SCREEN - 10	UR 8
☐ ORP	O.R. PANEL - 1ML WHOLE BLOOD HEPARINIZED RUSH TO LAB ON ICE	4						☐ AMP	AMPHETAMINES	UR
☐ ELC	ELECTROLYTES	G4	1,3					☐ BAR	BARBITURATES	UR
☐ NA	SODIUM	G2	3					☐ BNZ	BENZODIAZEPINE	UR
☐ K	POTASSIUM	G2	3		**MICROBIOLOGY X6361**			☐ THC	CANNABINOIDS	UR
☐ GAS	BLOOD GASES - 1ML WHOLE BLOOD, HEPARINIZED, RUSH TO LAB ON ICE			☐ GRM	GRAM STAIN			☐ CCN	COCAINE	UR
☐ CA	CALCIUM	G2	3	☐ STN	AFB STAIN (ONLY)			☐ OPT	OPIATES	UR
☐ CAI	IONIZED CALCIUM	G3	3	☐ INK	INDIA INK			☐ PCP	PCP	UR
☐ MG	MAGNESIUM	G2	3							
☐ GLF	GLUCOSE	G2	3							
☐ ACN	ACETONE	R2								
☐ CRT	CREATININE	G2	3		**DRUG MONITORING X6365**					
☐ BUN	UREA - N	G2	3	☐ ALD	ALCOHOL, ETHYL	R2				
☐ OSM	OSMOLALITY	G2	3	☐ DIG	DIGOXIN	R2				
☐ MBL	NEONATAL BILIRUBIN	RM	5	☐ LTH	LITHIUM	R3				
☐ CPK	CREATINE KINASE(CK)	R3		☐ PHE	PHENOBARBITAL	R2				
☐ CMB	CK-MB	R3		☐ DIL	PHENYTOIN (DILANTIN)	R2				
☐ AST	AST (SGOT)	G2	3	☐ SAL	SALICYLATES	R2			**TIMED URINE COLLECTIONS**	
☐ AMN	AMMONIA	L5	6	☐ THE	THEOPHYLLINE	R2			MO DAY TIME	
☐ AML	AMYLASE	R3						BEGUN		
☐ UAM	U. AMYLASE	UT							MO DAY TIME	
☐ SFG	CSF GLUCOSE	C 0.5						ENDED		
☐ SFP	CSF PROTEIN	C1			**ENDOCRINOLOGY X6365**			LAB USE:		
				☐ CGI	HCG, URINE	UR				
				☐ PGA	AMNIOSTAT, PG, QUAL	AF1			TOTAL TIME HR	
				☐ FLM	FETAL LUNG MATURITY - S/A LEVEL	AF2				
	HEMATOLOGY X6375			☐ CGB	HCG, BLOOD	R3			VOLUME ML	
☐ CCS	BLOOD CELL PROFILE	L5		☐ CGF	HCG, BLOOD FULL TITER	R3				
☐ PLT	PLATELET COUNT	L5							NOTES AND SPECIMEN	
☐ CBC	COMPLETE BLOOD COUNT (CCS and PLT)	L5							REQUIREMENTS - SEE REVERSE	
☐ CBD	CBC WITH DIFFERENTIAL	L5							**LAB USE ONLY**	
☐ PTT	ACTIVATED PARTIAL THROMBOPLASTIN TM	B5						ACCN NO.		
☐ PT	PROTHROMBIN TIME	B5								
☐ COS	COAG SURVEY	A B5 L5	7							
☐ FIB	FIBRINOGEN QUANTITATIVE	B5						LAB ID		

//// STAT //// STAT //// STAT //// STAT //// STAT //// STAT ////

OTHER TESTS - WRITE IN. CALL LAB IN ADVANCE TO ENSURE THAT TESTS WRITTEN IN CAN BE RUN STAT

0488-00 (1/91)

figure **11-2** Sample test requisition form. (Courtesy of Thomas Jefferson University Hospital Clinical Laboratories, Philadelphia, PA.)

NOTES

1. ELECTROLYTES INCLUDE:
   SODIUM
   POTASSIUM
   CHLORIDE
   CO_2

2. CHEM-7 PANEL CONSISTS OF:
   ELECTROLYTES
   UREA-N
   CREATININE
   GLUCOSE

3. THE LABORATORY WILL ACCEPT
   SERUM, HOWEVER WE CAN REPORT
   RESULTS ON A MORE TIMELY
   BASIS WITH PLASMA.

4. OR PANEL CONSISTS OF:
   BLOOD GASES
   SODIUM
   POTASSIUM
   IONIZED CALCIUM

5. PROTECT FROM LIGHT.

6. RUSH TO LAB ON ICE.

7. COAGULATION SURVEY
   INCLUDES PT, PTT, AND CBD.

8. DRUG SCREEN-10 INCLUDES TESTS FOR:
   AMPHETAMINES   METHADONE
   BARBITURATES   METHAQUALONE
   BENZODIAZEPINE   OPIATES
   CANNABINOIDS   PCP
   COCAINE   PROPOXYPHENE

SPECIMENS

AF — AMNIOTIC FLUID

B   — BLUE TOP TUBE (ALWAYS FILL TUBE)

C   — CEREBRO SPINAL FLUID

G   — GREEN TOP TUBE

L   — LAVENDER TOP TUBE

R   — RED TOP TUBE

UR — URINE, RANDOM

RM — MICROTAINER, RED TOP (ALWAYS FILL)

UT — URINE, TIMED

–   NUMBER FOLLOWING LETTER
    CODE INDICATES MINIMUM
    AMOUNT OF SPECIMEN
    IN ML.

figure **11–2** *Continued* Reverse side of form.

UNCOLLECTED SPECIMEN NOTICE THOMAS JEFFERSON UNIVERSITY HOSPITAL CLINICAL LABORATORIES	ROOM No.

PATIENT'S NAME

TEST(S)

Specimens requested were not collected because:

☐ Patient not in room - Call Lab to re-schedule

☐ Patient uncooperative _____

☐ Unable to draw _____

☐ Other: _____

COLLECTOR	TIME ☐a.m. ☐p.m.	DATE

LA-T-1

figure **11-3** Sample uncollected specimen notice. (From Laboratory Information Handbook. Philadelphia, Thomas Jefferson University Hospital Clinical Laboratories, September, 1991, p. 10.)

Whether performed by the laboratory or by the manufacturer, phlebotomy QC may include one of the four procedures listed in Table 11-4 and discussed in the text that follows.

Evaluating Evacuated Test Tubes. The purpose of evaluating evacuated test tubes is to measure the amount of vacuum draw and compare it with expected results under standard test conditions. A 1-m piece of flexible vinyl or latex tubing is connected to the tip of a 50-ml buret. A 20-gauge blood collection needle is attached to the open end of the tubing. The procedure continues by filling the buret with water, bleeding the air out of the tubing and needle, refilling the buret to bring the meniscus to "0," inserting the needle into the stopper of an evacuated tube, opening the stopcock of the buret, pushing the needle through the stopper, and allowing the tube to draw completely. The tube is then elevated so that its meniscus is at the same height as the buret meniscus (Fig. 11-5). The stopcock is closed, and the volume drawn from the buret is recorded (to 0.1 ml). Each tube for which the tested draw does not fall within ±10% of the labeled draw is defective.

Evaluating the Stopper Assembly. The purpose of evaluating the stopper assembly is to ensure that it will function as expected during

CAPILLARY SPECIMEN REQUIREMENTS

Pediatric specimens are accepted for a number of tests. This section lists all the common ones for which pediatric specimens can be used, and indicates the number of Microtainer blood tubes which are needed. This list is classified by general test type, i.e., chemistry, hematology, and so forth. Most specimens are serum (red top Microtainer), however please note that some require EDTA (lavender top tube).

Specimen amounts apply where the hematocrit of the patient is normal. If the hematocrit is high, it is suggested that the amounts shown be doubled.

	NUMBER of MICROTAINER(S)	COLOR
CHEMISTRY		
Acid Phosphatase	2	Red
Albumin	1/3	Red
Alkaline Phosphatase	2/3	Red
ALT	2/3	Red
Amylase	1/3	Red
AST	2/3	Red
Bilirubin (Fractionated)	1/2	Red
Calcium	1/3	Red
Chem-7 Panel (SMA7)	1	Red
Chloride	1/3	Red
Cholesterol	1/3	Red
CO_2	1/3	Red
Complement C3, C4	1	Red
CK	2/3	Red
CK Isoenzymes	1	Red
Creatinine	1/3	Red
Enzymes	1	Red
GGT	2/3	Red
Glucose	1/3	Red
Health Screen-12 (SMA 12)	1	Red
Immunoelectrophoresis	1	Red
Immunoglobulins	1	Red
LD	2/3	Red
LD Isoenzymes	1	Red
Lipase	1	Red
Magnesium	1/3	Red
Microbilirubin	1/2	Red
Osmolality	2/3	Red
Phosphate	1/3	Red

figure **11-4**   Sample pediatric specimen requirements. (From Laboratory Information Handbook. Philadelphia, Thomas Jefferson University Hospital Clinical Laboratories, September, 1991, p. 87.)

collection and sample mixing. Evacuated vacuum tubes are filled with water using a 20-gauge blood collection needle and holder. While the tube is removed slowly from the needle/holder, the stopper is examined to make sure it does not pull out of the tube. After placing the tube in a mechanical mixer and mixing for 20 minutes, the stopper is observed for overall looseness and leakage of water at the puncture point or around

table **11-4** **PHLEBOTOMY QC PROCEDURES**

1. Evaluation of evacuated test tubes
2. Evaluation of stopper assembly
3. Centrifuge test
4. Additive test

VACUUM DRAW

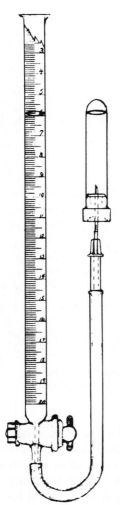

figure **11-5** Method for evaluating the amount of vacuum draw in evacuated test tubes. (Reproduced with permission from H1–A3, "Evacuated Tubes for Blood Specimen Collection—Third Edition; Approved Standard," NCCLS, 771 E. Lancaster Avenue, Villanova, PA 19085.)

the tube's rim. Stoppers that pull out, fall out, have general looseness, or leak during the steps of this test procedure are defective.

Centrifuge Test. In the centrifuge test, the ability of an evacuated tube to withstand the centrifugation needed to separate whole blood into its components is evaluated. After the vacuum tubes are completely filled with water, they are placed in centrifuge carriers, following the centrifuge manufacturer's directions. The tubes are spun for 10 minutes with a 2200 relative centrifugal force. Tube breakage of any degree indicates a defect.

Additive Test. The additive assay determines the quantity and identity of the chemical (e.g., anticoagulant) added to the evacuated tube. Assays follow United States Pharmacopeia (USP) or other appropriate chemical methods.

More detailed instructions for any of these QC procedures can be obtained from the National Committee for Clinical Laboratory Standards (NCCLS)[9] (771 East Lancaster Avenue, Villanova, PA, 19085; telephone, (215) 525-2435).

Perceptions of Quality

Delivering the right product/service (e.g., collection of blood specimens); satisfying the customer's needs; meeting the customer's expectations; and treating every customer with integrity, courtesy, and respect are the perceptions of quality in phlebotomy. Who are the customers of a phlebotomist? Patients are not the only customers; doctors, nurses, and other departments' employees are also customers.

What are the needs of these customers? Regardless of the customer, the basic need is assistance in detecting or treating an illness. All customers expect a relatively painless venipuncture, proper timing, clear instructions, use of proper technique, adherence to standard operating procedure (consistency), efficiency, effective interpersonal communication skills, and teamwork. Customers do not want or expect additional stresses. They want to be treated with integrity, courtesy, and respect. Using the best venipuncture technique means nothing to the customer who has been mistreated (e.g., yelled at, forced or coerced to permit testing, lied to, given false hopes, made the recipient of prejudice, etc.). Professional behavior is a key to quality patient care.

It is important to remember that phlebotomists are usually the only representative of the clinical laboratory who have direct patient contact. Patients, doctors, nurses, and others who have had an unpleasant experience with a phlebotomist are likely to have a negative image of the laboratory and its ability to provide quality services. However, the converse is also true. Positive experiences tend to yield positive patient outcomes. Members of a phlebotomy team can be considered the laboratory's public relations officers. Therefore, a laboratory QA program might include customer satisfaction surveys and incident report monitoring.

At times, extraneous situations arise that can interfere with quality work. Examples include, but are not limited to, patients who are being resuscitated, patients with traumatic injuries, combative patients, uncooperative family members, belligerent doctors or nurses, and frequent experiences of heavy workload and low staffing. Each of these, or any combination, tend to be stressful for the phlebotomist.

When these extraneous situations occur, effective coping tactics are needed. "All employees need to short-circuit negative emotions, especially anger, and achieve a level of calmness, clarity, and peace that lets them perform at their best." [10] Maintaining focus, adhering to standard operating procedures and referring to the manual when questioned, practicing assertive behaviors (neither aggressive nor passive), and being empathetic and professional will enable phlebotomists to handle these stressful occasions with pride and a positive outcome.

PROGRAM DESIGN AND IMPLEMENTATION

Knowing the aspects (e.g., skill, technique, timeliness, QC, supplies) and the perceptions (e.g., customer approval) of phlebotomy quality allows a laboratory to design a phlebotomy QA program unique to its facility. Recognizing which of these aspects and perceptions are high volume, high risk, high cost, and problematic provides additional direction in plan design and development. Indicators can be identified and thresholds established.

After deciding which of these key indicators should be monitored, data can be gathered and analyzed at a frequency suitable to the department. Employees are involved in data gathering, and usually, supervisory personnel summarize the data, analyze it, and pose courses of corrective action when thresholds are reached or exceeded. Corrective action may include steps such as employee retraining, contacting a supplier or service representative, notifying a clinical service, or modifying an existing procedure. After execution of corrective action, data gathering and analysis continues. Determining the appropriateness of the corrective action taken may require gathering and evaluating many months of data. As mentioned earlier, the employees using the supplies and performing the procedures are among the best sources of data and information. Depending on the aspect of care being studied, this process may never end.

Any time an incident occurs that might have an effect on customer perception or specimen quality, it should be reported to the appropriate laboratory supervisor. This information may help the laboratory diagnose problematic areas. These areas may eventually be included in the phlebotomy QA plan. Incorporation into the QA plan means that these areas (indicators) will be monitored, and the effectiveness of the corrective action taken will be evaluated.

Monitoring and evaluating patient care services also include reporting the findings to the appropriate persons (i.e., the department's employees, the department supervisor, and other top administrative officials within the organization). Inspectors from government and accrediting agencies will also want to review the QA reports. They will scrutinize corrective action documentation and the effectiveness of those actions in assuring quality patient care.

As mentioned previously, the focus of quality in health care is shifting from assurance to improvement. Fixing or correcting problems is no longer sufficient; instead, preventing them from happening and continuously striving for improvement is becoming central to quality patient care.

SUMMARY

A phlebotomy QA program is designed by combining the aspects and perceptions of blood collection quality with the JCAHO recommendations for monitoring and evaluating patient care services. Positive patient outcomes are the goal of any health care delivery service. Using and referring to the procedures in the specimen collection manual and reporting problems to supervisory personnel are important to assuring quality. The number and types of specimens rejected, the number of specimens recollected, the number of duplicate draws, the number of collection attempts, the number of specimens drawn from newborn and pediatric patients, incidents of untimeliness, and cases of customer complaints are usually the indicators included in a phlebotomy QA plan. Factors contributing to poor-quality services are sought and analyzed; corrective action is taken, when indicated; and the effectiveness of this action is studied.

Each employee's involvement in the entire process is fundamental to a successful QA plan. Monitoring and evaluating quality is a time-consuming process. However, the benefits (positive outcomes, satisfied customers, improved teamwork, improved profitability, etc.) are worth the investment and are important to an organization's survival.

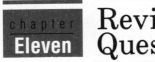

Review Questions

1. The values prompting study of an important aspect of care are called _____.
2. Evaluating vacuum tubes is a form of phlebotomy _____.
3. _____ are one of the best sources of data or information.
4. In the near future, _____ will become the focus of health care quality.
5. The process of monitoring, evaluating, and correcting patient care problems is called _____.

References

1. McBeth S: Continuous quality improvement: The Joint Commission perspective. Clin Lab Sci 5:87–89, 1992.
2. Hunt VD: Quality in America: How to Implement a Competitive Quality Program. Homewood, IL, Business One Irwin, 1992.
3. Garofalo VM, Rudmann SV: Clinical laboratory quality assurance: An overview. Clin Lab Sci 2:28–31, 1989.
4. College of American Pathologists, Commission on Laboratory Accreditation: General Laboratory Inspection Checklist. Northfield, IL, CAP, 1989–1990.
5. American Association of Blood Banks: Accreditation Requirement Manual. Arlington, VA, American Association of Blood Banks, 1989.
6. Joint Commission on Accreditation of Healthcare Organizations: Accreditation Manual for Hospitals. Chicago, Joint Commission on Accreditation of Healthcare Organizations, 1987.
7. Joint Commission on Accreditation of Healthcare Organizations: Monitoring and Evaluation in Support Services. Oakbrook Terrace, IL, Joint Commission on Accreditation of Healthcare Organizations, 1990.
8. Stewart CE, Koepke JA: Basic Quality Assurance Practices for Clinical Laboratories. Philadelphia, JB Lippincott, 1987, p 17.
9. National Committee for Clinical Laboratory Standards: Evacuated Tubes for Blood Specimen Collection. 3rd ed. Document H1–A3. Villanova, PA, NCCLS, 1991.
10. McCutchen G: Total quality people. Clin Lab Sci 5:94–95, 1992.

chapter Twelve

Medicolegal Issues and Health Law Procedures

Shirley E. Greening

The term "medicolegal" describes the interrelationship of the professions of law and medicine. The medicolegal field is sometimes called "medical law" or "legal medicine." Early medical law most often concentrated on **forensic medicine,** or the presentation of medical data or evidence in courts of law. Medical law has now expanded to encompass such fields as pathology, psychiatry, toxicology, public health regulation, health care legislation, court rulings, and administrative regulation of medical professional practice and medical service programs. Health law is a specialty area of law that relates to practitioners in medicine, dentistry, nursing, hospital administration, environmental health and safety, and allied health. The allied health professions include those individuals who work in laboratories located in hospitals, public health facilities, private or commercial enterprises, and research settings.[1]

Phlebotomists, as members of the laboratory health care team, are in a unique position in relation to most other laboratory personnel. In many health care settings phlebotomists may be the only laboratorians who come into face-to-face contact with patients or blood donors; they are the only laboratorians who perform specimen collection procedures on patients or donors, and the only laboratorians who deal with the very real issues of fear of infection, illness, and death and dying from the patient's perspective. Phlebotomists must have a strong educational background and good training; be technically proficient; follow laboratory procedures; be in compliance with government rules and regulations; and at the same time be good listeners, good communicators, and good public relations representatives. If phlebotomists become inattentive to, careless about, or unaware of their professional roles and duties, they may increase the risk of errors in the practice of their profession and thus increase the risk of being held legally liable for those errors. Examples of the most common errors are injury to a blood donor, misidentification of a patient, a mistake in interpreting a physician's orders, or transmission of disease.

Phlebotomists practice their profession at a time when patients and clients have high expectations for the success of their health care. Patients and clients are increasingly likely to question the quality of care or to object to treatments or procedures that they have perceived as harmful, injurious, or damaging to them. One result of this questioning may be that the patient or client takes legal action by filing a malpractice **claim** against the health care institution, the laboratory, and any individuals involved in their care, including phlebotomists.[2,3]

Another result may be that government regulatory agencies or laboratory accreditation organizations may call into question the way that a laboratory supervises its personnel or the ways in which a laboratory ensures that it is providing quality services and care to patients and clients.

Phlebotomists should be familiar with the various legal principles and the regulatory framework that affect their activities as members of the health care team. Phlebotomists should not conduct their professional activities in constant fear of legal liability (what some have termed "defensive medicine"). Rather, an understanding of why and how medicolegal issues arise in the day-to-day performance of phlebotomists' duties is part of phlebotomy education and practice.

SOURCES OF LAWS

Common law consists of those principles and rules of action that derive their authority solely from usages and customs that have evolved from ancient, unwritten laws of England. The common law is all the statutory and case law background of England and the American colonies before the American Revolution and is distinguished from statutory or legislative law, which developed after the American Revolution. Many common law principles have been incorporated into more formalized bodies of law governing cities, states, and nations.

Statutory law (also called "legislative law") is the body of law that is developed and promulgated by the United States Congress or by a state legislature as an outcome of the political process or societal influences. Legislatively enacted laws are called "statutes." A municipality may also enact laws, which are usually called "codes" or "ordinances."

Administrative law (also called "regulatory law") is not technically a set of laws, but instead consists of the rules and regulations that are written by government agencies to implement statutes or public laws. The United States Congress delegates authority to a variety of government agencies that then write the specific provisions of the statutes in a process know as **rulemaking.** Most agencies also have the power to monitor compliance with these rules and enforce penalties for noncompliance. In contrast to courts or legislatures, government agencies employ and consult with experts having special knowledge about the areas covered by statutes. Agencies also have much greater flexibility than courts or legislatures to revise regulations in response to social and economic changes or new scientific information. Courts or legislatures may defer to a government agency for an interpretation of a court rule or legislative statute.[4]

Decisional law (also called "case law") develops as a result of federal, state, or local courts deciding cases brought by two or more individual parties. Cases are decided based on precedents (a decision in a previous case), which can then be narrowed, expanded, distinguished, or overruled. Case law that is decided "once and for all" is termed *stare decisis;* if an issue had been litigated before by the same parties and cannot be litigated again, it is termed *res judicata.*[5] Case law can become statutory law where local, state, or federal government legislatures vote to incorporate a judicial line of decisions into the form of a statute. By passing legislation, governments recognize that decisions in individual cases have importance and application to all citizens.

Each source of law or method of law-making (statutory, case, and administrative) may deal with civil laws, criminal laws, or laws of equity. *Civil laws* are those that relate to private rights and remedies sought by citizens through proceedings termed civil actions. Civil actions are brought to enforce, redress, or protect an individual's private rights. *Criminal laws* (also termed "penal laws") refer to those state and federal statutes that define criminal offenses and specify corresponding penalties, fines, and punishments for offenses against the safety and welfare of the public or wrongs committed against the federal government or a state government. Criminal laws generally apply to misconduct that is willful, intentional, wanton, or reckless. The doctrine of *equity* was developed to administer justice on principles of fairness, especially when a court or an administrative agency does not have the power or the legal precedents to make, carry out, or enforce a decision.

Standards of proof in cases brought before regulatory, civil, or criminal forums are variable and can overlap depending on the severity and extent of a violation. For example, most questions regarding regulatory law are decided based on whether there was substantial compliance with an agency's rule or regulation. In a civil action, a plaintiff must show that it was more probable than not that a defendant caused an injury or other type of harm. Most criminal cases require that evidence of guilt be beyond a reasonable doubt.

AREAS OF LAW APPLICABLE TO PHLEBOTOMY PRACTICE

The phlebotomist's interactions with patients, clients, and other health care professionals can be viewed from different legal perspectives. Health care workers (most commonly physicians) and patients could be viewed as having an implied contractual relationship. A contract is formed when the physician offers or makes available health services, and the patient agrees to the medical care. The contract is formalized when the physician is paid. There is no requirement for an express written agreement between these two parties to the contract—the actions undertaken by the physician and patient essentially imply that a contract has been made. However, the physician-patient relationship thus formed is more than a mere business deal; it is a voluntary arrangement most aptly seen as creating a status or relationship rather than a contract. The physician-patient relationship gives rise to certain professional duties and **fiduciary** obligations even when there is no payment for services.[6]

A physician or a patient could be in breach of contract if either does not meet his or her part of the agreement. However, it is rare indeed for a physician to take legal action against a patient for not following medical instructions. In health law, it is overwhelmingly the patient who sues a physician, hospital, or health care worker. Why do patients sue? Because they believe the health professional has failed to do something that he or she should have done. This failure to meet a **standard of care,** when the health professional has a duty of due care to a patient, most commonly falls under the area of law known as *torts.* For a variety of reasons, claims against health care personnel are usually framed in terms of tortious conduct rather than breach of contract. Patients do not claim that a physician or other health care worker violated a contract; they claim that he or she committed a tort.[7]

A tort (from the Latin word *torquere,* meaning twisted) is a civil wrong or injury, other than breach of contract, that may be remedied by a court in the form of an action for damages. All torts involve a violation of some duty that is owed by one individual to another individual. When phlebotomists, a phlebotomy service, or a laboratory employing phlebotomists is held liable for an injury or other damage to a patient or client, each may be blamed for intentionally or unintentionally acting, or failing to act, in a manner that caused an injury. The patient or client who claims to be injured is called the **plaintiff.** The person being blamed is the **defendant.**

Intentional Torts

In the context of health care, claims falling under the category of intentional torts usually arise in conjunction with questions about whether a patient gave permission for or consented to a medical procedure, a treatment, or a diagnostic test. When these circumstances occur, they are generally framed as a charge of *assault* or *battery.* In most jurisdictions, assault and battery are criminal offenses.

Assault is any active, willful attempt or threat to inflict injury on another person that is coupled with an apparent ability to inflict such harm. Assault can be committed without actually touching or striking; it is the plaintiff's sense of awareness and apprehension of imminent harm that determines whether there is an assault. Assault is often defined as an unlawful attempt to commit a battery.

Battery can be viewed as an active intent to cause harm or injury to a person without that person's consent that actually does harm the person. The offer or threat to use harm is an assault; the use of it is battery. Because battery always includes an assault, the two are commonly combined in the phrase "assault and battery." The term "technical battery" is sometimes used to describe those situations in which a physician or other health care worker, in the course of treatment, exceeds the consent given by the patient even though no harmful purpose was intended.

When a patient enters a hospital or a client comes into a blood-drawing center, the presumption is that he or she has consented to be treated or has consented to be a donor. However, few individuals would give blanket consent to any and all possible medical procedures without being given more information with which to make an informed choice. (See "Consent and Informed Consent.") If a phlebotomist proceeds to collect blood after a patient has refused to have blood drawn, the patient could claim that the act of the phlebotomist approaching him or her with a needle was an assault. If the act of drawing blood was perceived by the patient as painful or injurious, he or she could claim that a battery was committed.

It is not uncommon for patients to feel stress when confronted with medical decisions and procedures. However, occasionally the behavior of health care personnel can intentionally or unintentionally produce severe emotional reactions in patients. Intentional behavior (conduct or words) that is particularly outrageous and extreme can lead to a charge of intentional infliction of emotional distress. Even if conduct is not intended to threaten, if the patient perceives a threat, he or she may claim negligent infliction of emotional distress. Obviously, the phlebotomist must avoid threatening language ("if you don't let me draw blood, you're going to die") or gestures (acting out a painful procedure) that could create such distress.

Unintentional Torts

When a health care worker violates a duty owed to a patient or client, it is called "malpractice." Malpractice can be defined as professional misconduct, an unreasonable lack of skill in or faithfulness to professional duties, illegal or immoral conduct, ignorance, or neglectful or careless mistreatment that leads to injury, unnecessary suffering, or death of a patient or client. Most legal actions involving malpractice by health care personnel are grounded in the theory of **negligence,** the failure of a "duty of due care."

NEGLIGENCE: WHAT MUST BE PROVED?

In every legal action for negligence, the plaintiff must go through a four-step process to prove that a health care worker is at fault for failing to perform some legal duty. These four steps, called "elements," are duty, breach of duty, causation, and damages.

Plaintiffs have the burden of proving each of these four elements. In most malpractice cases, if even one element cannot be proved, then the defendant is not held liable for malpractice. However, in some instances an average reasonable person who has no special professional knowledge could conclude that an injury would not have occurred in the absence of a negligent act. When a breach of duty is obvious to a layperson, the doctrine of *res ipsa loquitur* ("the thing speaks for itself") can be applied. This has the effect of shifting the **burden of proof** to the defendant, who must then prove that he or she was *not* negligent.

Duty. As a citizen, every individual has a duty to behave as a reasonably careful person would, given the same or similar circumstances. This standard of behavior means that individuals must act or refrain from acting so as not to injure or damage another person or that person's property. The duty to meet a standard of behavior or care can arise from a state statute or city ordinance (e.g., "Do not cross the street when the light is red"). In health care, duty is usually established by standards of care or practice that exist by custom or by professional rules and guidelines. The legal standard of care is ". . . that degree of skill, proficiency, knowledge and care ordinarily possessed and employed by members in good standing in the profession . . ." The standard has to be shown to exist, and the phlebotomist must be performing in the capacity applicable to that standard.

Those persons engaged in professions that require special knowledge and skills are judged according to a standard of care upheld by similar professionals. For the phlebotomist, the test to determine what he or she did or should have done would be, "What would a reasonable, prudent phlebotomist have done under the same or similar circumstances?" In the past, physicians and other health professionals were held to standards that existed in their own communities (the so-called locality rule). Because health professionals now have access to information outside of their own communities, this standard has been expanded to include what would be expected in similar communities. When national standards exist, such as national certification examinations or national accreditation standards for schools, a national standard of care can be imposed. This is true for the profession of phlebotomy—for example, a phlebotomist in California would be held to the same standard of care used for a phlebotomist in New York.

Breach of Duty. Conduct that exposes others to an unreasonable risk of harm is a breach of duty. The plaintiff must be able to show what actually happened and that the defendant acted unreasonably. Either **direct** or **circumstantial evidence** can demonstrate what happened. If the defendant knew or should have known that there was a reasonable probability that his or her conduct would cause harm, then the defendant will be found to have breached the duty of due care.

Causation. The cause of harm or injury is both a factual and a legal question. To show *cause-in-fact* (or actual cause), the plaintiff must demonstrate that he or she would not have been injured but for the conduct of the defendant. There must be a direct line from the conduct to the injury, with no intervening circumstances and no other factors or events that contributed to the injury. "Proximate cause" is the term used to distinguish legal causation from factual causation. Legal (proximate) cause is a policy choice that essentially determines who should bear the costs of harm. If an injury was reasonably foreseeable by the defendant, then the defendant will be held legally liable for the injury.

Damages. Once negligence and causation are established, plaintiffs must be able to show that they were actually damaged by the negligent act. The harm to a plaintiff may be physical, emotional, or financial. In these circumstances, courts attempt to place a monetary value on the injury. Compensatory damages attempt to reimburse the plaintiff to the position the plaintiff was in before he or she was injured. Special damages allow recovery of economic losses during the time of injury, which may be for medical bills or lost wages, but can also be for future losses. Future losses might include the costs of continuing medical treatment or loss of future wages if the person is unable to return to work. General damages are those costs related to the injury itself. Punitive damages, those assessed to punish a defendant, are usually not awarded in negligence cases, unless the defendant's conduct was reckless or willful.

LIABILITY OF EMPLOYERS FOR PHLEBOTOMY PERSONNEL

Most phlebotomists are employed by hospitals, independent laboratories, or other health care organizations, and when a phlebotomist is found to be negligent, his or her employer can also be found negligent. The employer, employee's supervisor, or a laboratory director may be vicariously liable when the employee's negligent conduct falls within the scope of the employment, regardless of whether the employer was actually present or had the ability to control the employee's conduct. *Respondeat superior* ("let the master answer") is the legal doctrine that places an employer in a position of responsibility for the acts of its employees. An employer has an affirmative duty to control the conduct of employees.

In corporate negligence theory, a hospital, its board of directors, administrators, and reviewing committees, and any other persons who act as agents for the corporation owe a duty of due care to patients. The principles of corporate negligence are similar to those of vicarious liability, but in corporate negligence, liability is imposed on the corporate entity and on nonmedical agents of the corporation, rather than on negligent physicians or allied health personnel. Examples of corporate negligence include a hospital's hiring an unqualified laboratorian, or a hospital's maintaining an unsafe environment for patient treatment.

The types of duties owed by a hospital directly to a patient include a duty to use reasonable care in maintaining safe and adequate equipment and facilities, a duty to oversee all who practice medicine within the hospital walls, a duty to select and retain competent physician and non-physician personnel, and a duty to establish and enforce policies and rules that ensure quality care for patients.[8] Under corporate liability, a hospital cannot avoid liability by delegating these duties to physicians or other individuals who work in the hospital.

How Is the Phlebotomy Standard of Care Determined?

Courts and plaintiffs rely on a variety of sources to show that standards of care and practice exist for a particular profession. All states have statutes called "Medical Practice Acts" (MPAs) that define the qualifications and experience necessary to legally practice medicine. MPAs usually delineate which medical procedures or tests can be delegated to other health personnel under a physician's supervision, and they prohibit anyone who is not licensed as a physician or other health professional (such as a nurse or physical therapist) from practicing healing or diagnostic medicine. State licensing boards generally review cases in which a person is engaged in the unauthorized practice of medicine. MPAs are enforced through disciplinary actions imposed by licensing boards and, in extreme cases, by criminal sanctions.[9]

Many states also *license* allied health personnel. Because most state licensing boards require some proof of qualification for licensure, lack of a license may be used to demonstrate a failure to meet a standard of care. Situations may arise in which a person has the appropriate education, training, or experience to practice in an allied health profession but does not have a license to practice. When an individual is not licensed and malpractice is shown, that individual's conduct may be declared to be **negligence per se,** in which practicing without a license is a violation of a statute.[5]

Hospital and laboratory *certification or accreditation standards and guidelines* can be used to demonstrate quality control and quality assurance procedures in phlebotomy practice. Even when standards are voluntary, compliance with or awareness of standards and guidelines can be used to show that a phlebotomy service or a phlebotomist knew or should have known what procedures and conduct were appropriate under the circumstances. Certification and accreditation guidelines are especially effective as **evidence** of practice standards when they are applicable nation-wide and followed by a wide variety and number of phlebotomy services and phlebotomy practitioners. Examples of organizations that accredit or certify phlebotomy services include the Joint Commission on Accreditation of Healthcare Organizations (JCAHO), the College of American Pathologists (CAP), and the American Association of Blood Banks (AABB).

Mandatory standards in the form of federal, state, and local laws and regulations are commonly used to establish a statutory standard of practice for phlebotomy services. Regulations usually outline minimum standards of performance. Mere compliance with a statutory requirement does not necessarily protect phlebotomy services and personnel from negligence actions, especially if it can be shown that personnel knew or should have known that more comprehensive actions were required, either in general or as related to the specific circumstances surrounding the plaintiff. Examples of federal statutory standards are those contained in the Clinical Laboratory Improvement Amendments of 1988 (CLIA '88)[10] and the Occupational Safety and Health Administration's (OSHA's) Rules on Occupational Exposure to Bloodborne Pathogens.[11] States may have health and safety statutes that are similar to or more stringent than federal standards. Cities usually have health and safety codes or ordinances that govern areas such as storage of chemicals and disposal of waste materials. When both federal and state laws or regulations apply to laboratory practice, the laboratories are usually required to abide by whichever of the laws is more stringent.

Statements of competencies, such as those contained in the National Accreditation Agency for Clinical Laboratory Sciences' (NAACLS) Phlebotomy Programs Approval Guide,[12] or designated responsibilities such as those listed in the National Phlebotomy Association (NPA) Guidelines[13] describe tasks and skills required of phlebotomy practitioners. These can be used to show how an individual failed to meet a particular level of performance. For example, if there is a question as to whether the phlebotomist performed a capillary collection correctly and the competency expects an entry-level phlebotomist to be able to perform the correct procedure for capillary collection, the statement of competency can be used to establish the appropriate standard of care in that situation.

Professional practice guidelines, which appear in brochures or bulletins written or endorsed by professional organizations, can be used to show a recommended practice that is viewed by the profession as clinically effective or technically superior. Guidelines may relate to timing of blood collections, collection of patient data, preservation and handling procedures, or follow-up and documentation protocols.

Technical guidelines and standards that describe how to perform a certain test or procedure can be used to show how a phlebotomist was negligent in the collection, handling, or transportation of blood specimens.[14]

Scientific journals and textbooks *(learned treatises)* can be used to demonstrate that knowledge was available to a practitioner at the time of the negligent act, thereby showing what the practitioner should have known or done.

The **testimony** of expert witnesses is commonly used to establish the standard of practice in a health profession. In a case involving a phlebotomist, an experienced phlebotomist, a physician, or a phlebotomy supervisor can be asked to state an opinion on what constitutes acceptable quality control or assurance practices.

OTHER LEGAL DOCTRINES AND AREAS OF LAW APPLICABLE TO PHLEBOTOMY PRACTICE

Interplay Among the Rights of Privacy, Confidentiality, and Informed Consent

The issues litigated in legal disputes involving intentional and unintentional injury to patients and clients by health care workers have their roots in guaranteed individual rights. These rights have their basis in the United States Constitution and Bill of Rights, regardless of whether they are specifically enumerated in the Constitution. For example, the U.S. Constitution does not mention a right of privacy; however, the United States Supreme Court has recognized that a right of privacy exists and that certain areas of privacy are guaranteed under the Constitution.[7] The right of privacy includes the right to confidentiality, and if this right is waived, consent to the waiver must be informed.

Right of Privacy. An individual's right "to be let alone," recognized in all United States jurisdictions, includes the right to be free of "intrusion upon physical and mental solitude or seclusion" and the right to be free of "public disclosure of private facts."[7] Every health care institution and health care worker has a duty to respect a patient's or client's right of privacy, which includes the privacy and confidentiality of information obtained from the patient/client for purposes of diagnosis, medical records, and public health reporting requirements. If a health care worker conducts tests on or publishes information about a patient/client without that person's consent, the health care worker could be sued for wrongful invasion of privacy, **defamation,** or a variety of other actionable torts.

Confidentiality. Health care workers must be vigilant in keeping information about patients and clients confidential. This is especially true in blood banks, transfusion services, and phlebotomy services, where phlebotomists may have access to information about patients who are human immunodeficiency virus (HIV)–positive, have acquired immuno-deficiency syndrome (AIDS) or other sexually transmitted diseases, or who may have medical histories that, if disclosed, might cause undue embarrassment to or prejudice or discrimination against that patient. Phlebotomists and their supervisors should understand that they have a legal duty to keep records, documentation, and laboratory test results confidential. This duty may be waived only if a patient has given express permission for the information to be released, if the patient has sued the institution or its health care personnel, or if the health care worker is specifically obligated to release patient information (e.g., to the Centers for Disease Control and Prevention or other authorized public health department). Even in the last situation, care must be taken to ensure that the confidentiality of patient records and reports cannot be breached while they are being communicated or are in transit.[9]

Consent and Informed Consent. Physicians and other health care workers are required to obtain a patient's consent before performing any invasive or diagnostic procedure. Consent can take a variety of forms (e.g., written agreements, spoken words, implicit actions, or making an appointment for a test). In a nineteenth century case, for example, a plaintiff's failure to object to a vaccine that the defendant was preparing to give to the plaintiff conveyed apparent consent to the injection.[15]

However, to agree to a medical procedure, a patient must first know what he or she is agreeing to. Thus, the doctrine of consent has expanded to include *informed consent,* which emphasizes that health care workers must fully disclose any risks, alternatives, and benefits of a procedure or test so that the patient/client can make an informed decision about whether he or she wants to be treated or tested.[16] "[T]he doctrine of informed consent imposes on a physician, before he subjects his patient to medical treatment, the duty to explain the procedure to the patient and to warn him of any material risks or dangers inherent in or collateral to the therapy, so as to enable the patient to make an intelligent and informed choice about whether or not to undergo such treatment."[17]

The correlate to informed consent is *informed refusal.* Patients may refuse treatment for religious, social, financial, or other reasons, but even in these cases a health care worker may be found negligent for the lack of information given to the patient, if the patient didn't have enough information available to make a reasonable decision to forego treatment.[16]

In general, it is the physician who has the duty to disclose adequate information to a patient. Phlebotomists should be wary of volunteering information to a patient in situations where they do not have the legal or professional authority to do so. These situations may be difficult "judgment calls" for the phlebotomist, as patients often ask phlebotomists questions about their treatment or why they are drawing blood. The phlebotomist should politely refer the patient to his or her physician or charge nurse for these explanations.

Patient's Bill of Rights

In the early 1970s, the American Hospital Association developed a policy statement for health care institutions and their patients that incorporated and reflected the individual rights guaranteed under the legal doctrines of privacy, informed consent, and confidentiality. Since that time, many hospitals have adopted the *Patient's Bill of Rights* into their policy manuals, and some state legislatures have passed Patient's Bill of Rights statutes.[18]

The *Patient's Bill of Rights* is intended to "promote the interests and well-being of the patients and residents of health care facilities."[1] As such, it enumerates the patient's right to respectful care, to adequate information with which to make an informed decision (or refusal) about his or her care, and to confidentiality in treatment and communication of records about his or her medical care program. In addition, the document affirms a patient's right to information about medical bills and charges, possible involvement in medical research and experimentation, and hospital rules and regulations (see Table 9–2).

Medical Devices and Equipment Failures

Phlebotomists use many pieces of equipment or reagents that are manufactured by medical equipment or pharmaceutical companies and then purchased by the hospital or laboratory from manufacturers, distributors, or retailers. These supplies — whether they be needles, syringes, protective equipment or clothing, chemicals, or blood — may, in unusual situations, be defective or unsafe because of the way they were designed, assembled, or screened, or they may be inherently dangerous even when used under normal conditions. When a patient suffers a needle break during blood drawing, has a violent reaction to a drug, or contracts an infectious disease after use of a product, he or she may sue the manufacturer of that product under various legal theories, including negligence, strict liability in tort, and breach of *implied warranty of merchantability*.

Under negligible theory, plaintiffs must prove that defendants have a duty to conform to certain standards of care in the manufacture of their products and to guard against unreasonable risks. *Strict liability in tort* is imposed when manufacturers are held liable for injuries caused by an unreasonably dangerous or defective product, even if there is no finding of fault. Breach of an implied warranty of merchantability may be found, on the basis that manufacturers or sellers of goods should be obligated to provide consumers with products that are fit for the purpose for which they are being sold.

These legal actions fall under the law of *products liability*. Products liability focuses on the liability of suppliers for defective products that cause physical harm. The defect in question may not be the actual product itself; defects may arise because of inadequate packaging, instructions, or warning labels.[19]

The term "product" implies goods that are sold predominantly in commercial settings. Manufacturer liability for defective health care products has received much professional and legal attention, because health care treatment and diagnostic testing has traditionally been viewed as a service rather than as a product. Especially in the areas of blood transfusions (which may result in HIV transmission) and genetically engineered pharmaceuticals (such as coagulation components), the distinction between products and services has been challenged by plaintiffs who sue blood banks or pharmaceutical companies to recover damages resulting from transmission of infectious diseases.

Because the availability of blood and blood products is of great importance to public health, many states have passed blood shield statutes that exempt blood transfers, blood derivatives, or blood products from the threat of products liability lawsuits and specifically mandate that blood components are to be considered medical services, not goods or products. **Immunity** from legal action thus guarantees an adequate blood supply for use in medical emergencies and treatment of chronic blood-related disorders.

CASE LAW

As the range of health care services has expanded and health care personnel have become more specialized, the reach of malpractice **litigation** is no longer confined to the physician-patient relationship and may include nonmedical personnel as part of the health care team. Although most of the following cases did not specifically involve phlebotomists, the situations in which these claims arose can be readily analogized to laboratory and phlebotomy practice. These cases do not represent an exhaustive review of phlebotomy-related malpractice but are intended to remind phlebotomists of problems that may develop when practice standards and procedures are compromised.

Belmon v St. Frances Cabrini Hospital, 427 So2d 541, 544 (LaApp, 1983) [Negligent blood sample collection by a medical technician caused hemorrhage.]

Butler v Louisiana State Board of Education, 331 So2d 192, 196 (LaApp, 1976) [A donor fainted and sustained injuries, and a biology professor was held negligent for not giving students previous instructions on blood drawing and donor care.]

St. Paul Fire and Marine Insurance Co v Prothro, 590 SW2d 35 (Ark App 1979) [Negligent physical therapy procedures caused a patient to develop a *Staphylococcus* infection.]

Simpson v Sisters of Charity of Providence, 588 P2d 4 (Or 1978) [Radiology technician performed a poor-quality radiograph that failed to demonstrate a fracture that subsequently caused paralysis.]

Southeastern Kentucky Baptist Hospital, Inc v Bruce, 539 SW2d 286 (Ky 1976) [Misidentification of a patient led to a surgical procedure on the wrong patient.]

Wood v Miller, 76 P2d 963 (Or 1983) [Negligent use of diathermy equipment burned a patient.]

Favalora v Aetna Casualty and Surety Co, 144 So2d 544 (La App 1962) [A patient fainted and fell, causing injuries; a radiology technician and supervising physician were found negligent for not being alert to and prepared for the patient's condition.]

McCormick v Auret (Ga 1980) [Failure to use sterile equipment during venipuncture led to nerve damage secondary to infection.]

Alessio v Crook, 633 SW2d 770 (Tenn App 1982) [Failure to include an x-ray report in the patient's medical record before patient discharge resulted in more extensive surgery than would have been required had the physician seen the report.]

Variety Children's Hospital v Osle, 292 So2d 382 (Fl App D3 1974) [A surgeon failed to label and separate specimens sent to a pathology laboratory. Because the pathologist was unable to determine which of the two specimens was malignant, removal of both of the patient's breasts was necessary.]

Jeanes v Milner, 428 F2d 598 (Ark 1970) [A 1-month delay in mailing specimens to a laboratory resulted in delayed diagnosis of cancer; if it had been detected promptly and treated, the pain and suffering of the patient could have been lessened.]

Ray v Wagner, 176 NW2d 101 (Minn 1970) [A patient claimed a physician was negligent for failing to timely notify her of her malignancy; the patient was found contributorily negligent for giving the physician incomplete and misleading information about how she could be reached.]

Thor v Boska, 113 Cal Rptr 296 (1974) [A physician's inability to produce medical records after he had been sued for malpractice created an inference of guilt.]

Lauro v Travelers Insurance Company, 262 So2d 787 (La App 1972) [A hospital was not negligent for not using the latest laboratory equipment available, where current standards of care demonstrated that the equipment used was acceptable.]

DEFENSES TO LEGAL CLAIMS

If faced with a lawsuit brought by a patient, the laboratory and the phlebotomist may resort to several defenses to avoid a finding of liability.

Statutes of Limitation

All states have statutes of limitation that restrict or limit the length of time in which a claimant can file a cause of action after an injury. The purpose of statutes of limitation is twofold; first, they are intended to compel legal actions within a reasonable time so that potential litigants have a fair opportunity to defend themselves while evidence and witnesses are still available.[7] Second, they allow presumably innocent parties to continue their lives and livelihoods without the constant and continuing threat of liability.

In malpractice cases, statutes of limitation can start at several points: at the time of the negligent act, at the time when the injury was discovered; or when the physician-patient relationship ends.

The length of time these statutes run varies from state to state and can be as little as a few months to many years, depending on the cause of action and nature of the injury. Statutes of limitation may also be *tolled* (suspended or stopped temporarily) if, for example, the plaintiff is a child, the defendant is absent from the jurisdiction, or the injury in question has been fraudulently concealed.

Contributory Negligence

In rare malpractice situations, a patient's own actions may fall below the standard to which a reasonably prudent patient might be expected to conform. For example, if a patient, during the course of a routine blood collection procedure, unreasonably manipulates or otherwise interferes with the venipuncture to the extent that he or she is injured, and then sues the phlebotomist for the injury, the phlebotomist may raise the affirmative defense of contributory negligence.[20]

In some states, contributory negligence completely bars recovery against the defendant, even if the defendant is found negligent. In other states, a finding of contributory negligence has the effect of reducing the amount of monetary damages against a negligent defendant.

Adequate and Accurate Records as the Best Defense

The importance of detailed, legible, comprehensive record keeping and documentation for laboratory procedures and patient identification cannot be overemphasized. Documentation relating to the laboratory not only is required by federal regulations and accreditation organizations, it is also essential in the legal arena. Legal action against a laboratory rarely takes place at the moment malpractice occurs; claims may be filed years later; and even after a claim is filed, it may be several more years before all evidence is collected in the **discovery** process, and the claim is litigated in court. During this waiting period, memories fade, contemporaneous records may be misfiled or lost, and laboratory personnel change.

Laboratory notations and records should never be altered or changed without documentation of the reasons for the change. Indeed, poorly maintained, sloppy, or altered records may prejudice a jury against a laboratory or health care professional, no matter how well intentioned the change might have been.

A laboratory's or phlebotomist's best defense is the ability to produce witnesses and records that substantiate adherence to acceptable professional standards of practice for documenting identifiable specimen collection, test procedures, test reporting, records storage and archiving procedures, quality control and quality assurance methods, and remedial or corrective actions when laboratory errors occur.[7]

Chain of Custody in the Clinical Laboratory

Chain of custody is a rule of legal evidence that requires an authorized person (e.g., police officer, attorney, clinical or forensic testing laboratory, or medical examiner) to account for the location, control, and integrity of a specimen, result, or report at all times. Any break in this chain of custody, from specimen collection to the presentation of test results in a court of law, may suggest that the specimen was tampered with or otherwise altered. If continuous and uninterrupted custody cannot be established, the laboratory specimen may not be admissible as evidence in a legal case.[21]

It is not uncommon for phlebotomists to be called on to collect urine or blood specimens from individuals for the purpose of screening for narcotics, alcohol, or infectious agents. Phlebotomists may also be required to transport specimens that may become evidence in a criminal investigation. To establish each link in the chain of custody, each component step of the specimen testing process (including requisition and report forms) must be documented. Most often this is accomplished by a chain-of-custody form that accompanies the specimen. All individuals who receive, release, or otherwise come into contact with the specimen are required to sign, date, and time-stamp the form to show that the specimen was not tampered with. Phlebotomists or other laboratory workers may be asked to testify about their role in maintaining the chain of custody.

Although the primary purpose of establishing a chain of custody is to ensure that evidence is admissible, the documentation required is not unlike the quality and accuracy-based patient test management provisions of CLIA '88 (see later). In legal cases alleging patient misidentification, lost specimens, or missing reports, laboratories may be required to show not only an unbroken chain of custody, but also that they have complied with the provisions of CLIA '88.

LEGAL AND PROFESSIONAL PROTECTIONS FOR THE PHLEBOTOMIST

Many of the legal doctrines and statutory provisions covered in this chapter focus on the rights and protections available to patients, clients, and donors when faced with substandard or negligent laboratory and phlebotomy practices. Phlebotomists, too, may be concerned about their own exposure to hazardous or infectious agents or about unsafe working conditions. Phlebotomists do have recourse to address these concerns, in addition to bringing unsafe conditions to the attention of their immediate supervisors.

When phlebotomy services are understaffed, phlebotomists are sometimes called on to perform additional tasks that are either beyond the scope of their expertise or increase workloads to the point at which patient care is compromised. Especially in the area of nursing, *Protest of Assignment Forms* are sometimes used as a means to alert supervisors to potentially dangerous practice situations. These forms usually become part of the employee's file and therefore should not be used casually or merely to complain about a short-term situation. They should be used by the phlebotomist only when an extra work assignment is protracted, excessive, clearly unreasonable, and imminently dangerous to the phlebotomist or to his or her patients.

The regulations of the Occupational Safety and Health Administration, and analogous state agencies, are specifically designed to protect the health and safety of employees in the workplace. Phlebotomists should report any hazardous or unsafe materials, conditions, or practices to their supervisor and should be active participants in the formulation of workplace policies to avoid or protect against these situations.

It is generally not necessary for phlebotomists to purchase individual professional liability (malpractice insurance) policies, as most health care employers and institutions cover employees under blanket policies. Phlebotomists should check to see whether they are specifically included in or excluded from the employer's insurance policy and whether their employer's policy is an "occurrence" or "claims-made" policy. Occurrence policies protect employees even at a future date, provided that the policy was in effect at the time when the malpractice incident occurred. A claims-made policy is one that must be continually in force at both the time of the incident and the time the claim is made.

Phlebotomists who are self-employed, either as temporary workers placed in positions through an employment agency, or as independent contractors, may purchase professional liability insurance through several companies that provide individual or group coverage to allied health practitioners. Liability policies usually cover monetary damages for personal injuries up to preset limits and usually include coverage for attorney fees and court costs. Many companies provide legal counsel as part of the coverage.

REGULATION OF LABORATORIES AND LABORATORY PRACTITIONERS

In the past few years, laboratories, laboratory practitioners, and other health care workers have been subject to heightened scrutiny and oversight by state and federal government agencies, both for the protection of the health and welfare of the public and for their own protection. Although state laboratory regulation is quite diverse, federal regulation is intended to apply to virtually all laboratory and health care settings.

Clinical Laboratory Improvement Amendments of 1988

In October 1988, the U.S. Congress passed Public Law 100-578, CLIA '88, amid a flurry of television and newspaper coverage about some poorly run laboratories that were misdiagnosing or mishandling laboratory tests, and reports of questionable business and payment practices of other laboratories. Congress delegated authority to administer this public law to the Health Care Financing Administration (HCFA). The HCFA, within the U.S. Department of Health and Human Services (DHHS), is the agency that administers the federal government's medical reimbursement and health care payment programs, Medicare and Medicaid.

The federal regulations implementing CLIA '88 went into effect on September 1, 1992. They are intended to ensure the quality and accuracy of laboratory testing by creating a uniform set of provisions governing all laboratories that examine human specimens for the diagnosis, prevention, or treatment of any disease or impairment of, or the assessment of the health of, human beings.[10] Virtually every clinical testing laboratory in the United States, whether in a hospital, a physician office laboratory, or an independent facility, must be certified by the federal government. Facilities that only collect or prepare specimens (or both) or only serve as a mailing service and do not perform testing are not considered laboratories.

Laboratories are subject to inspections by federal and state agencies. Government inspectors or their agents can periodically review laboratory operations to ensure compliance with CLIA '88.

Under CLIA '88, the level of regulatory oversight and performance expectations is dependent on the complexity of a given test procedure, rather than on the location or type of laboratory. All laboratory tests (called "analytes") are categorized as waived, moderately complex, or highly complex, with highly complex testing subject to the most stringent regulations. The level of test complexity is determined by assessing the relative simplicity or difficulty of conducting the test and the relative risk of harm to the patient if the test is performed incorrectly.

The CLIA '88 regulations include provisions for preanalytical, analytical, and postanalytical steps in the testing process. Regulations mandate proficiency testing of laboratories based on the types of test they perform. In addition, laboratories are required to demonstrate and document their quality control and quality assurance procedures, to ensure that patient tests and records are managed appropriately, and to demonstrate that testing personnel have adequate education, training, and experience to perform tests. The focus of the CLIA '88 regulations is on *outcome measures* — laboratories must show that the methods used to test specimens lead to accurate, reliable, quality test results.

Laboratories not meeting the conditions required by the CLIA '88 provisions can be subject to various sanctions and penalties. These range from directed plans of correction to withholding of payment from the Medicare and Medicaid programs for laboratory tests. Laboratories that remain out of compliance with the regulations may be shut down or have substantial monetary fines imposed.

Phlebotomists are responsible for performing many of the pre- and postanalytical steps in the blood testing process. The laboratory's overall performance and its ability to maintain consistent and reproducible quality tests rely in large part on the quality and preservation of specimens collected by the phlebotomist. Therefore, knowledge of and compliance with these provisions can not only contribute to quality patient care, but also provide the phlebotomist and the laboratory with some measure of protection against regulatory sanctions and civil lawsuits.

The following selected provisions of CLIA '88 have special significance to phlebotomists and phlebotomy practice.

Subpart J: Patient Test Management

§493.1101 Condition. Each laboratory performing moderate or high complexity testing, or both, must employ and maintain a system that provides for proper patient preparation; proper specimen collection, identification, preservation, transportation, and processing; and accurate result reporting. This system must ensure optimum patient specimen integrity and positive identification throughout the preanalytic (pretesting), analytic (testing), and postanalytic (post-testing) processes and must meet the standards of this subpart as they apply to the testing performed.

§493.1103 Standard; Procedures for specimen submission and handling

(a) The laboratory must have available and follow written policies and procedures for each of the following, if applicable: methods used for preparation of patients; specimen collection; specimen labeling; specimen preservation; conditions for specimen transportation; and specimen processing. Such policies and procedures must ensure positive identification and optimum integrity of patient specimens from the time the specimens are collected until testing has been completed and the results reported.

(c) Oral explanation of instructions to patients for specimen collection, including patient preparation, may be used as a supplement to written instructions where applicable.

§493.1105 Standard; Test requisition.
The laboratory must perform tests only at the written or electronic request of an authorized person. . . . The laboratory must ensure that the requisition or test authorization includes

(a) The patient's name or other unique identifier;

(b) The name and address or other suitable identifiers of the authorized person requesting the test and, if appropriate, the individual responsible for using the test results or the name and address of the laboratory submitting the specimen, including [the name of] a contact person;

(c) The test(s) to be performed;

(d) The date of specimen collection; . . . and

(f) Any additional information relevant and necessary to a specific test to ensure accurate and timely testing and reporting of results.

§403.1107 Standard; Test records.
The laboratory must maintain a record system to ensure reliable identification of patient specimens as they are processed and tested to assure that accurate test results are reported. These records must identify the personnel performing the testing procedure. . . . The record system must provide documentation of information, including

(a) The patient's identification number, accession number, or other unique identification of the specimen;

(b) The date and time of specimen receipt into the laboratory;

(c) The condition and disposition of specimens that do not meet the laboratory's criteria for specimen acceptability.

§493.1109 Standard; Test report

. . . (a) The laboratory must have adequate systems in place to report results in a timely, accurate, reliable, and confidential manner and to ensure patient confidentiality throughout those parts of the total testing process that are under the laboratory's control. . . .

(e) The results or transcripts of laboratory tests or examinations must be released only to authorized persons or the individual responsible for using the test results.

Subpart K: Quality Control

§493.1201 General quality control . . . (b) The laboratory must establish and follow written quality control procedures for monitoring and evaluating the quality of the analytical testing process of each method to ensure the accuracy and reliability of patient test results and reports.

§493.1204 Standard; Facilities. The laboratory must provide the space and environmental conditions necessary for conducting the services offered [including space, ventilation, utilities, and safety precautions for protection against physical hazards and biohazardous materials].

§493.1205 Standard; Test methods. The laboratory must utilize test methods, equipment, instrumentation, reagents, materials, and supplies that provide accurate and reliable test results and test reports.

§493.1211 Standard; Procedure manual

(a) A written procedure manual for the performance of all analytical methods used by the laboratory must be readily available and followed by all laboratory personnel.

§493.1215 Standard; Equipment maintenance and function checks. The laboratory must perform equipment maintenance and function checks that include electronic, mechanical, and operational checks necessary for the proper test performance and test result reporting of equipment, instruments, and systems. . . .

§493.1221 Standard; Quality control records. The laboratory must document and maintain records of all quality control activities . . . for at least two years. . . . In addition, quality control records for blood and blood products must be maintained for a period not less than five years after processing records have been completed or six months after the latest expiration date, whichever is the later date. . . .

Subpart M: Personnel

§493.1423 Standard; Testing personnel qualifications. Each individual performing moderate complexity testing must

(a) Possess a current license issued by the State in which the laboratory is located, if such licensing is required; . . . and

(4) (i) Have earned a high school diploma or equivalent; and

(ii) [Have documentation of training that ensures the individual has the skills required for proper specimen collection, including patient preparation, if applicable, labeling, handling, preservation or fixation, and processing or preparation; for performing preventive maintenance and troubleshooting . . . ; a working knowledge of reagent stability and storage; and an awareness of factors that influence test results.]

Phlebotomists should note that although their specific duties and functions within their work setting may place them outside the scope of personnel standards for the purposes of federal CLIA '88 regulations, the laws of the state in which their workplace is located may have more specific phlebotomy requirements. Therefore, the personnel standards listed above are intended only to provide a general outline.

Subpart P: Quality Assurance

§493.1701 Each laboratory . . . must establish and follow written policies and procedures for a comprehensive quality assurance program that is designed to monitor and evaluate the ongoing and overall quality of the total testing process. . . . The laboratory's quality assurance program must evaluate the effectiveness of its policies and procedures; identify and correct problems; assure the accurate, reliable, and prompt reporting of test results; and asssure the adequacy and competency of the staff. As necessary, the laboratory must revise policies and procedures based on the results of those evaluations. . . . All quality assurance activities must be documented.[10]

Other Regulatory Agencies Governing Laboratories and Phlebotomists

Many state and federal laws and agencies govern laboratory practice in some way. Employment practices, wages and salaries, business practices, facilities construction, intra- and interstate transportation of specimens, licensing of personnel, and testing methodology are but a sampling of laboratory-related government oversight activities that affect the clinical laboratory. Although a complete listing of these agencies is beyond the scope of this chapter, listed below are the federal agencies, apart from the Health Care Financing Administration, that have substantial influence on laboratories in the United States.[22,23]

The Occupational Safety and Health Act of 1970 established the *Occupational Safety and Health Administration* (OSHA) within the U.S. Department of Labor. The OSHA is the federal agency that sets rules and regulations covering all aspects of employer and employee safety and health. This agency sets workplace standards and regulates such areas as ventilation; noise; fire and electrical safety; labeling and appropriate precautions for flammables; biologic chemical, and radiation hazards; and safe exposure levels.

The *Food and Drug Administration* (FDA) is responsible for the approval of virtually all medical and diagnostic equipment, devices, pharmaceuticals, reagents, and diagnostic tests before they can be marketed for sale and used in health care settings. The FDA, through its process of premarket approval and its content-labeling requirements, has evaluated the safety, clinical efficacy, and medical need of almost all the testing equipment, reagents, and supplies used by the phlebotomist.

The *Centers for Disease Control and Prevention* (CDC), through its various offices and divisions, serves as a federal resource for developing technical and scientific standards and conducting epidemiologic, health and safety, quality assurance, and health evaluation and proficiency studies and programs.

The *Environmental Protection Agency* (EPA) monitors and enforces regulations for the safe disposal of chemical and other hazardous wastes, including biologic hazards.

The *U.S. Postal Service* has developed regulations covering the safe packaging and transport of human biologic specimens through the mails and requires appropriate warning labels to protect postal workers from potentially hazardous or infectious agents.

Importantly, almost all of these agencies or departments (i.e., OSHA, FDA, CDC, HHS) have some level of oversight over transfusion services and blood banks, in addition to general laboratory oversight.

SUMMARY

The ability to demonstrate sound laboratory management principles and compliance with regulatory provisions, professional accreditation guidelines, and practice standards can provide substantial protection against the threat of litigation. No laboratory or health care worker can be completely protected from lawsuits, but potential liability can be minimized by conscientious and continuous attention to good laboratory practice.

Review Questions

1. The federal agency responsible for approving and regulating medical devices, pharmaceuticals, and diagnostic test kits is the _____.
2. The legal responsibility of an employer for the negligent acts of employees is called _____.
3. The legal doctrine of _____ requires that a patient must be able to make an intelligent and reasoned decision about whether or not he agrees to a medical procedure or diagnostic test.
4. Imposition of liability on manufacturers for defective blood and blood products falls under the law of _____.
5. When a patient who has filed a lawsuit has disregarded a physician's orders or acts unreasonably, thus causing all or part of the injuries sustained, the defendant may use the defense of _____.

References

1. Curran WJ, Hall MA, Kaye DH: Health Care Law, Forensic Science, and Public Policy. 4th ed. Boston, Little, Brown, 1990.
2. Peterson RG: Malpractice liability of allied health professionals: Developments in an area of critical concern. J Allied Health 14:363–372, 1985.
3. Oliver R: Legal liability of students and residents in the health care setting. J Med Educ 61:560–560, 1986.
4. Gelhorn E, Boyer BB: Administrative Law and Process: In a Nutshell. 2nd ed. St. Paul, MN, West Publishing, 1981.
5. Black MA: Black's Law Dictionary. 5th ed. (abridged). St. Paul, MN, West Publishing, 1983.
6. Havighurst CC: Health Care Law and Policy: Readings, Notes, and Questions. Westbury, NY, The Foundation Press, 1988.
7. Wadlington W, Waltz JR, Dworkin RB: Law and Medicine: Cases and Materials. Mineola, NY, The Foundation Press, 1980.
8. *Thompson v Nason Hospital*, 591 A2d 703 (Pa 1991).
9. Furrow BR, Johnson SH, Jost TS, Schwartz RL: Health Law: Cases, Materials and Problems. 2nd ed. St. Paul, MN, West Publishing, 1991.
10. Department of Health and Human Services, Health Care Financing Administration, Public Health Service: 42 CFR 405 *et seq*, 57 *FR* 7002-7186, February 28, 1992.
11. Department of Labor, Occupational Safety and Health Administration: Occupational exposure to bloodborne pathogens. 29 CFR 1910.1030; 56 *FR* 64004-64182, December 6, 1991.

12. National Accrediting Agency for Clinical Laboratory Sciences: Phlebotomy Programs Approval Guide. Chicago, NAACLS 1986.
13. National Phlebotomy Association: Guidelines. Washington, NPA, 1980.
14. National Committee for Clinical Laboratory Standards: Procedures for the Collection of Diagnostic Blood Specimens by Skin Puncture. 2nd ed. Code H4-A2, Villanova, NCCLS, 1986; Collection, Transport, and Preparation of Blood Specimens for Coagulation Testing and Performance of Coagulation Assays. NCCLS Document H21-A. Villanova, NCCLS, 1986; Procedures for the Domestic Handling and Transport of Diagnostic Specimens and Etiologic Agents. 2nd ed. Code H5-A2. Villanova, NCCLS, 1985.
15. *O'Brien v Cunard,* 28 NE 266 (Mass. 1891).
16. Swartz M: The patient who refuses medical treatment: A dilemma for hospitals and physicians. Am J Law Med 11:147–194, 1985. See also *Truman v Thomas,* 611 P2d 902 (Ca 1980).
17. *Sard v Hardy,* 879 A2d 1014 (Md 1977).
18. American Hospital Association: Patient's Bill of Rights. Chicago, AHA, 1973.
19. Shapo MS: Products Liability: Cases and Materials. Mineola, NY, The Foundation Press, 1980.
20. *Smith v McClung,* 161 SE 91 (S. Ct. NC 1931).
21. Chamberlain RT: Chain of custody: Its importance and requirements for clinical laboratory specimens. Lab Med 20:477–480, 1989.
22. Wilcox KR, Baynes TE, Crable JV, et al: Laboratory Management. In Inhorn SL, ed: Quality Assurance Practices for Health Laboratories. Boston, American Public Health Association, 1978.
23. Rose SL: Clinical Laboratory Safety. Philadelphia, JB Lippincott, 1984.

Glossary

Activated Partial Thromboplastin Time   A coagulation test to monitor Factors I, II, V, VIII, IX, X, XI, and XII, often referred to as the intrinsic coagulation system.

Aerobic   A condition requiring the presence of oxygen.

Alveoli   Plural of aveolus; small air sacs in the lung where oxygen and waste products are exchanged with the blood.

Ambulatory   Able to walk; not bedridden.

Anaerobic   A condition in which oxygen is absent.

Analyte   Substance to be assayed.

Anticoagulants   Substances that prevent coagulation.

Attenuated   Made weak or made less able to cause disease.

Bacteremia   The presence of microorganisms in the blood.

Barrier Precautions   Protective clothing and other measures taken to prevent or reduce the chance of exposure to a disease-producing agent.

Basal State   A reference point with which test results are compared.

Burden of Proof   The obligation to affirmatively prove the facts of a disputed issue by the evidence presented.

Capital Equipment   Refers to equipment to be maintained indefinitely. Most institutions set a minimum price for equipment; anything costing more than that amount is considered capital equipment and requires special permission to purchase.

Carbon Dioxide   A waste product of metabolism consisting of one carbon atom and two oxygen atoms (CO_2), excreted primarily through the lungs.

Cardiac Muscle   The muscle of the heart.

CBC   Abbreviation for a complete blood cell count, which includes red blood cell count, white blood cell count, hemoglobin, hematocrit, mean corpuscular volume (MCV), mean cellular hemoglobin (MCH), mean cellular hemoglobin concentration (MCHC), and platelet count.

Claim   A demand for money or property, or a demand to assert one's own rights. In malpractice claims, an individual files a cause of action (which states the facts that the person believes give rise to a right to judicial relief) and claims an amount of money (damages) he or she believes will compensate him or her for injury.

Coagulation Factors   A series of proteins that, when activated, result in clot formation.

Conjunctivitis   Inflammation of the mucous membrane that lines the eyelids.

Convulsions   Involuntary muscular contractions and relaxations; can be caused by stress, hysteria, medication, neural defect, etc.

Corrective Action   An activity geared toward problem resolution.

Defamation   Holding a person up to ridicule, scorn, or contempt, or disrespect, which tends to injure that person's reputation. Defamation includes libel and slander.

Defendant   The person against whom recovery is sought in a lawsuit. In malpractice, the defendant can be a physician, hospital, allied health practitioner, or other health care provider.

Diabetes Mellitus   A disorder of carbohydrate metabolism caused by a lack of insulin and characterized by high blood glucose levels.

Diastole, Diastolic   The part of the heart beat cycle when the heart is in relaxation; normal diastolic range is approximately 60–80 mm Hg in healthy young adults.

Differential   A breakdown of the various types of white blood cells present in peripheral blood.

Discovery   The methods used to obtain facts and information about a case to assist in preparation for trial. In health law, discovery can include oral and written questions, asking for laboratory tests and results, requiring physical examination of patients, collecting medical records and documents, and interviewing witnesses.

Edema   The presence of an excessive amount of tissue fluid; may be localized or general.

EDTA   Abbreviation for the anticoagulant ethylenediaminotetraacetate.

Epidemiologic   Refers to factors that determine the frequency of disease and its distribution.

Etiologic   Refers to factors that cause disease.

Evidence   The facts and information about a case that are known, available, or collected through the discovery process and are used to persuade or convince a judge or jury.
    Direct evidence   Evidence in the form of testimony of a witness who actually saw, heard, or touched the subject under question.
    Circumstantial evidence   Evidence not based on actual personal knowledge that indirectly shows the facts to be proved.

Expired   As used in the text, synonymous with "deceased."

Femoral Vein   The major vein that runs on the upper, inner thigh of mammals.

Fiduciary   A person having a duty to act for another's benefit and in whose actions is placed another's trust, confidence, and faith.

Forensic Medicine   The application of every area of health care knowledge to the purposes and limits of the law.

Gonads   The sex organs: testes (male) and ovaries (female).

Hematoma   A swelling or collection of blood caused by a break in a vessel wall.

Hemoglobin   The substance contained in red blood cells that transports oxygen from the lungs to the tissues.

Hemolysis   The destruction of red blood cells.

Hemorrhage   Abnormal discharge of blood.

Hemostasis   Arrest of bleeding, thereby maintaining the integrity of the blood vessels and the blood flow.

Hormone   A substance secreted by a gland or organ that acts on another gland or organ. Examples are estrogen, progesterone, adrenalin, and testosterone.

Hypertension   High blood pressure.

Hypoglycemia   Abnormally decreased blood glucose level.

Hypovolemia   Decreased blood volume.

Immunity (legal)   Exemption from duties imposed by a law or from liabilities arising from a law.

Indicators   Specific, measurable variables of important aspects of care.

Infectious   Pertaining to a disease caused by a microorganism that may be transmitted to another person.

Inventory   A list of supplies that is updated as supplies are used.

Jargon   As it is used in a laboratory, terms or expressions that may not be understood by individuals unfamiliar with a clinical laboratory.

Jugular Vein   The major vein that runs on either side of the trachea, and the major venipuncture site in animals.

Lactic Acid   A waste product generated from the breakdown of glycogen during muscle activity.

Lipemia   The presence of an abnormally large amount of lipids (fat) in the circulating blood.

Litigation   A lawsuit, including all the proceedings occurring before, during, and after a trial.

Lymph   A generally clear, colorless fluid that contains protein, water, and lymphocytes.

Maculopapular   A skin eruption consisting of discolored spots or patches on the skin that are not raised or depressed, combined with solid, red, raised eruptions that resemble pimples.

Mandible   The bone of the lower jaw.

Medial Saphenous Vein   A major vein that runs on the inner lower leg of mammals.

Metabolism   Physical and chemical changes produced in substances within the body.

Myasthenia Gravis   A disease characterized by great muscular weakness and progressive fatigability.

Negligence   Failure to do something that a reasonable person would ordinarily have done, or doing something that a reasonable person would not have done.

Negligence per se   The unexcused violation of a statute.

Neoplasms   Abnormal formation of tissue; tumors or growths that are harmful to the host.

Nosocomial   Infections acquired by patients while in the hospital.

Opportunistic Infections   Diseases caused by certain microorganisms that would otherwise be nonpathogenic, but, because of an altered physiologic state of the host, are given the opportunity to cause infection.

Osteomyelitis   Inflammation of bone, usually caused by a pathogenic organism.

Oxygen   An element that is essential to most forms of plant and animal life.

Palpate   To feel or touch.

Pathogen   A microorganism or substance that is able to produce disease.

Percutaneous   Through the skin.

Permucosal   Through the mucous membranes.

Phlebotomy   The surgical opening of a vein to collect blood.

Plaintiff   The person who brings a legal action or lawsuit (also called a *complainant*).

Plasma   The clear fluid that collects at the upper half of a tube of centrifuged blood, consisting of serum and protein substances in solution.

Polycythemia Vera   A disease characterized by an increasing number of red blood cells and an increase in total blood volume.

Prophylaxis   Measures taken to prevent disease.

Prothrombin Time   A coagulation test to monitor Factors I, II, V, VII, and X, often referred to as the extrinsic coagulation system.

Quality   A degree of excellence.

Quality Assurance   The process of making sure standards of care have been maintained by detecting, monitoring, evaluating, and correcting problems affecting patient care.

Quality Control   A process that (1) validates actual results by comparing them with expected results and (2) quantifies variations between the two.

Recurrent Tarsal Vein   The vein that runs on the inner surface of the guinea pig's lower leg.

Retro-orbital Plexus   The vein complex behind the inner portion of the eye.

Rulemaking   The process by which governmental agencies conduct research, consult experts, and draft regulations to implement laws passed by Congress or state legislatures.

Septicemia   An infection of the blood; the presence of pathogenic organisms in the blood.

Serum   The clear liquid portion of the blood without its fibrin and corpuscles.

Skeletal Muscle   Also known as voluntary or striated muscle; mainly composes the muscle that can be controlled.

Smooth Muscle   Also known as involuntary muscle; found primarily in the visceral organs.

Sphygmomanometer   An instrument to measure blood pressure.

Standard of Care   That degree of care, competence, or skill that a reasonably prudent person would exercise in the same or similar circumstances.

Stereotyping   Holding that all members of a given group can be characterized by simplistic guidelines.

Subordinate   A person whom you supervise.

Syncope   Fainting.

Systole, Systolic   The part of the heart beat cycle occurring when the heart is in contraction; normal systolic range is approximately 100–140 mm Hg in healthy young adults.

Tapped   Entered, penetrated (jargon).

Testimony   Evidence given by a witness under oath.

Threshold   Points/values that prompt the study of an aspect of care.

Vascular Implant   A surgically placed metal or plastic device by which blood can be removed for sampling.

WBC   White blood cell.

Answers to Chapter Review Questions

Chapter 1

1. Diagnosis
   Treatment
2. On the job
3. Physician office laboratories
   Blood collection centers
   Research institutes
   Veterinary offices
4. To ensure employers that the phlebotomists they hire meet a minimally acceptable standard of practice
5. American Society for Medical Technology

Chapter 2

1. Cell
2. System
3. Cardiac
4. Gonads
5. Platelets

Chapter **3**

1. Handwashing
2. Hepatitis B
3. Immune globulin
4. AIDS
5. Recap

Chapter **4**

1. EDTA
2. Lancet
3. Needles
4. Tourniquet
5. Splash guard

Chapter **5**

1. Patient identification
2. 70% Isopropyl alcohol
3. Tourniquet
4. Wash your hands and change your gloves
5. Strenuous exercise

Chapter **6**

1. Blood gases
2. 450 ml
3. Septicemia
4. Osteomyelitis
5. Sphygmomanometer

Chapter **7**

1. Petechiae
2. Hypovolemia
3. Edema
4. Hemolysis
5. Hematoma

Chapter **8**

1. Lavender-top
2. Serum
3. Jugular
   Cephalic
   Recurrent tarsal
4. Heart
   Ear
5. Eight to 12 hours

Chapter **9**

1. Life skills
2. Intrapersonal
3. Reference gap
4. Profession
5. Continuing education

Chapter **10**

1. True
2. To receive orders and to obtain patient information
3. Children
   Mentally retarded patients
4. Workload units
5. Goals
   Objectives

Chapter **11**

1. Thresholds
2. Quality control
3. Employees
4. Continuous quality improvement
5. Quality assurance

Chapter **12**

1. Food and Drug Administration (FDA)
2. Vicarious liability
3. Informed consent
4. Products liability
5. Contributory negligence

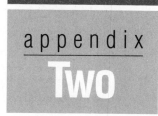

appendix
Two

Practice Examination for Certification

1. Blue-stoppered tubes are used primarily for the following assay:

   a. CBC
   b. Blood glucose determination
   c. Prothrombin time
   d. Rapid plasma reagin

2. Sodium heparin is the anticoagulant found in which of the following tubes?

   a. Blue
   b. Green
   c. Lavender
   d. Red

3. Yellow-stoppered tubes are used for:

   a. Blood cultures
   b. Compatibility testing
   c. Cholesterol assays
   d. WBC differential

4. The liquid portion of the blood collected from a red-stoppered tube after centrifugation is:

   a. Anticoagulant
   b. Plasma

215

    c. Serum

    d. Sodium citrate

5. A phlebotomy quality assurance program may include each of the following EXCEPT:

    a. Abnormal glucose quality control results

    b. Customer satisfaction surveys

    c. Number of hemolyzed specimens

    d. Number of mislabeled specimens

6. Which of the following is an aspect of quality?

    a. Delivering the right product/service

    b. Doing it right the first time

    c. Meeting the customer's expectations

    d. Treating every customer properly

7. Hemolysis is a reason for specimen rejection. It may be caused by all of the following EXCEPT:

    a. Clotting, because of insufficient mixing with the anticoagulant

    b. Introduction of alcohol used for cleaning the site into the vacuum tube

    c. Shaking the vacuum tube too vigorously when mixing

    d. Using a very small gauge needle and a large vacuum tube

8. All of the following procedures should be performed in the nursery when a phlebotomist collects a capillary specimen from an infant EXCEPT:

    a. Applying a bandage when bleeding has stopped to prevent infection

    b. Keeping a log of how much blood has been collected

    c. Wearing a gown and gloves

    d. Wiping away the first drop of blood

9. The order for filling tubes once blood has been collected in a syringe is:

    a. blue, red, green, yellow

    b. red, blue, yellow, green

    c. yellow, blue, green, red

    d. yellow, blue, red, green

10. The term that describes the interrelationship of law and medicine is:

    a. Forensic science
    b. Litigation
    c. Medicolegal
    d. Standard of care

11. Medical malpractice lawsuits are most often brought under the legal theory of:

    a. Contracts
    b. Criminal law
    c. Equity
    d. Negligence

12. Laws passed by the U.S. Congress are called:

    a. Cases
    b. Ordinances
    c. Regulations
    d. Statutes

13. The legal term for the intent to cause harm or injury to a person without the person's consent, and which actually does harm that person, is:

    a. Battery
    b. Breach of contract
    c. Negligence
    d. Product liability

14. When a patient refuses to have blood drawn, the phlebotomist should do the following EXCEPT:

    a. Contact the patient's nurse
    b. Force the patient to have blood drawn
    c. Return the requisition to the laboratory
    d. Try to convince the patient to have blood drawn

15. Technical errors causing no blood to be collected include:

    a. Missing the vein
    b. Needle goes through the vein
    c. No vacuum in the tube
    d. All of the above

16. Which of the following is not a reason for avoiding an area of the arm when performing venipuncture?

    a. Edema
    b. Obesity
    c. Petechiae
    d. Scarred veins

17. What is the first course of action if a patient has convulsions?

    a. Call for help
    b. Notify a physician
    c. Offer juice to help revive the patient
    d. Remove the tourniquet and needle

18. All of the following statements are true EXCEPT:

    a. Gray-stoppered tubes are used for blood glucose tests.
    b. Gray-stoppered tubes are used for CBC and WBC tests.
    c. Lavender-stoppered tubes are used for CBC, WBC, and platelet tests.
    d. Red-stoppered tubes are used for many tests, including serum enzyme tests.

19. Spurious laboratory results can be caused by:

    a. Hemolysis and lipemia
    b. Improper blood-to-anticoagulant ratio
    c. Improper handling of a sample during or after blood collection
    d. All of the above

20. Normally the serum produced after spinning blood in a red-stoppered tube is:

    a. Anticoagulated
    b. Clear or straw colored
    c. Milky white
    d. Pink

21. Which of the following is considered to be a noninfectious bodily substance according to the CDC guidelines known as the universal precautions?

    a. Amniotic fluid
    b. Blood
    c. Semen
    d. Tears

22. Which of the following diseases would require the use of respiratory precautions?

   a. Hepatitis B
   b. *Salmonella* infection
   c. Staphylococcal skin abscesses
   d. Tuberculosis

23. All of the following are vaccine-preventable diseases EXCEPT:

   a. AIDS
   b. Hepatitis B
   c. Polio
   d. Mumps

24. Which blood vessels generally carry blood that is high in oxygen?

   a. Arteries
   b. Veins
   c. Venules
   d. All are equally oxygenated.

25. Which system gives the body structure and protects vital organs?

   a. Integumentary system
   b. Muscular system
   c. Skeletal system
   d. Vascular system

26. The sebaceous glands are associated with the:

   a. Endocrine system
   b. Integumentary system
   c. Skeletal system
   d. Vascular system

27. All of the following may be required of a phlebotomist EXCEPT:

   a. Donor blood collections
   b. Injections
   c. Specimen preparation
   d. Therapeutic phlebotomies

28. Several items contribute to determining workload units. Which of the following DO NOT contribute to workload units calculations?

   a. Certification of phlebotomists
   b. Number of stat collections

    c. Size and number of hospital units

    d. Type of patients

29. Which collection round is routine in all hospitals?

    a. Early morning

    b. Late afternoon

    c. Mid-morning

    d. Noon

30. Which of the following is not an example of expendable equipment?

    a. Alcohol swabs

    b. Blood pressure cuffs

    c. Gloves

    d. Tubes

31. The standard operating procedure manual for specimen collection contains each of the following EXCEPT:

    a. Information on how to prepare the patient for the test

    b. Notes on timing requirements

    c. Specimen labeling requirements

    d. The laboratory supervisor's name and home telephone number

32. The quality of blood specimens is best summarized by which of the following statements?

    a. Phlebotomy technique is not critical to test results.

    b. Specimen handling has no effect on laboratory results.

    c. Specimens of low quality can produce inaccurate and potentially dangerous results.

    d. The laboratory will detect any problem with the specimens.

33. The glucose tolerance test:

    a. Is a monitor of blood glucose levels after ingestion of 300 gm of glucose

    b. Is performed to aid in the diagnosis of diabetes mellitus

    c. Lasts 1 hour

    d. May be collected in a blue-stoppered tube

34. The specimen for fibrin degradation products is collected in:

    a. A lavender-stoppered tube containing sodium citrate

    b. A syringe containing heparin

    c. A tube containing an enzyme inhibitor and thrombin

    d. A red-stoppered tube

35. The rule of legal evidence that requires documentation of the location and integrity of any laboratory specimens used as evidence in a trial is called:

    a. Accreditation
    b. Chain of custody
    c. Learned treatise
    d. Professional liability insurance

36. Policies adopted by some hospitals that incorporate the patient's constitutional rights to privacy, confidentiality, and informed consent in medical treatment are referred to as:

    a. Patient's Bill of Rights
    b. Protest of assignment forms
    c. Statutes of limitation
    d. Technical guidelines

37. When a hematoma is forming, all of the following are acceptable EXCEPT:

    a. Adjust the depth of the needle
    b. Ignore it and collect the specimen
    c. Remove the needle and apply pressure to the site
    d. Try another site

38. Technical errors causing a short draw include:

    a. A collapsed vein because of too much vacuum in the tube
    b. Lack of vacuum in the tube
    c. Placement of the needle bevel against the vessel wall
    d. The syringe plunger withdrawn too quickly

39. Hemoguard is a type of:

    a. Anticoagulant
    b. Lancet
    c. Needle
    d. Splash guard

40. A retractable sheath is part of a:

    a. Disposal container
    b. Lancet
    c. Multiple-draw needle
    d. Single-draw needle

41. Green-stoppered tubes may be used for all of the following laboratory tests EXCEPT:

    a. Ammonia
    b. CBC
    c. Chromosome analysis
    d. Human leukocyte antigen typing

42. Which of the following is not classified as a barrier precaution?

    a. HBV vaccine
    b. Gloves
    c. Goggles
    d. Gown

43. The most common cause of blood culture contamination is:

    a. Collection of too much blood
    b. Collection of the sample from below the intravenous line
    c. Improper skin preparation
    d. The use of a needle and syringe for collection

44. Nosocomial infections are:

    a. Acquired during a period of hospitalization
    b. Acquired in the womb before birth
    c. Symptomatic at the time of admission
    d. Transmitted by pets in the home

45. Which of the following viruses are transmitted primarily through contact with infected blood?

    a. Hepatitis A virus and rubella virus
    b. Hepatitis B virus and human immunodeficiency virus
    c. Influenza virus and human immunodeficiency virus
    d. Polio virus and hepatitis C virus

46. Which of the following are characteristics of a profession?

    a. Distinct field of knowledge
    b. Full-time occupation
    c. High degree of autonomy
    d. All of the above

47. Continuing education is:

    a. Formalized classroom study after high school that results in an academic degree

b. Education acquired from workshops and seminars attended after formal education has ended

c. Formal education resulting in a postbaccalaureate degree

d. None of the above

48. Which of the following cells contribute most to blood clotting?

a. Lymphocytes
b. Platelets
c. Red blood cells
d. White blood cells

49. Another name for erythrocytes is:

a. Lymphocytes
b. Platelets
c. Red blood cells
d. White blood cells

50. The tricuspid and bicuspid valves are associated with the:

a. Heart
b. Liver
c. Spleen
d. Stomach

51. The single most important step in phlebotomy is:

a. Cleansing the site
b. Patient identification
c. Using a clean needle
d. Using the proper evacuated tube

52. Which of the following is the vein of choice for venipuncture?

a. Basillic
b. Cephalic
c. Median cubital
d. Pulmonary

53. The bevel of the needle should be in which position before entering a vein?

a. Facing down
b. Facing toward the side
c. Facing upward
d. It really does not matter, as long as the venipuncture is performed quickly

54. Which of the following steps are in the proper order?

    a. Remove the needle, release the tourniquet, apply pressure
    b. Apply pressure, release the tourniquet, remove the needle
    c. Remove the needle, apply pressure, release the tourniquet
    d. Release the tourniquet, remove the needle, apply pressure

55. Which of the following IS NOT a physiologic condition that may cause variation in the basal state?

    a. Diet
    b. Exercise
    c. Gender
    d. Trauma

56. Striving for quality requires:

    a. Commitment
    b. Enthusiasm
    c. Time
    d. All of the above

57. As a quality-oriented phlebotomist, what would you do when encountering a combative patient?

    a. Attempt the venipuncture anyway; after all, you have a job to do
    b. Be empathic
    c. Immediately tie the patient to the bed rails or chair
    d. Play psychological games with the patient

58. When performing an arterial puncture, the phlebotomist should:

    a. Apply pressure on the site for 15 minutes after the collection
    b. Collect only from patients who have fasted for 12 hours
    c. Tie the tourniquet tight to obtain good blood flow
    d. Use the thumb to palpate

59. Medical screening for blood donors includes all of the following EXCEPT:

    a. Blood pressure
    b. Cholesterol
    c. Hemoglobin
    d. Weight

60. Therapeutic phlebotomy is performed as a treatment for patients with:

    a. Diabetes mellitus
    b. Hepatitis
    c. Lymphocytic leukemia
    d. Polycythemia vera

61. Blood smears:

    a. Are used to count red blood cells
    b. Are used to differentiate white blood cells
    c. Must be made from a drop of blood from a finger stick
    d. Should be made very slowly and carefully

62. Blood cultures MAY NOT be collected:

    a. Directly into aerobic and anaerobic culture bottles
    b. In a red-stoppered tube
    c. In a syringe
    d. In a yellow-stoppered tube

63. Which of the following is NOT one of the four elements that must be proved in a legal action for negligence?

    a. Analyte
    b. Breach of duty
    c. Causation
    d. Duty

64. A patient sitting in a chair has fainted. Possible acceptable actions by the phlebotomist include all of the following EXCEPT:

    a. Going quickly for help
    b. Placing a cold compress on the back of the patient's neck
    c. Putting the patient's head between the knees
    d. Using ammonium salts

65. All of the following will cause clotting in an anticoagulated tube EXCEPT:

    a. Blood collected in a syringe that is not added quickly to tubes with anticoagulant
    b. Hemolysis of red blood cells
    c. Improper blood-to-anticoagulant ratio
    d. Insufficient mixing of blood and anticoagulant

66. "The degree of skill, proficiency, knowledge and care ordinarily possessed and employed by members in good standing in the profession" is the legal definition for:

    a. Certification
    b. Damages
    c. Standard of care
    d. Testimony

67. Aspirin may affect a patient's:

    a. Bleeding time
    b. Blood cultures
    c. Blood gases
    d. Glucose level

68. When a patient is absent from his or her room, the phlebotomist should do all of the following EXCEPT:

    a. Check with the nurse to locate the patient
    b. Draw blood from the patient in a new location if possible
    c. Make a note on the requisition form if unable to collect the specimen
    d. Try to find the patient after lunch

69. Gloves should be worn:

    a. During all venipunctures and capillary punctures
    b. For HIV-positive patients only
    c. Only in cases of isolation
    d. Only when in the laboratory

70. The isolation or precaution category that would be the most important for phlebotomists is:

    a. Blood and body fluid precautions
    b. Enteric precautions
    c. Respiratory precautions
    d. Strict isolation

71. All of the following anticoagulants inhibit the clotting process by binding calcium EXCEPT:

    a. EDTA
    b. Potassium oxalate
    c. Sodium citrate
    d. Sodium heparin

72. Cytology is the study of:

   a. Cells
   b. Muscles
   c. Organ systems
   d. Tissues

73. The epidermis is a very important part of the:

   a. Cardiac system
   b. Integumentary system
   c. Nervous system
   d. Skeletal system

74. What is the substance in erythrocytes that carries oxygen?

   a. Albumin
   b. Glucose
   c. Hemoglobin
   d. Sodium chloride

75. An individual is considered Rh positive or negative depending on the presence or absence of:

   a. A Antigen on the red cells
   b. B antigen on the white cells
   c. D antigen on the red cells
   d. D antigen on the white cells

76. Which of the following is the primary source of information for labeling a specimen?

   a. Patient's nurse
   b. Patient's family
   c. What the patient tells the phlebotomist
   d. Patient's wristband

77. Which of the following is true about microcapillary collection?

   a. It is not necessary to wear gloves.
   b. One can usually collect as much blood as in venipuncture.
   c. The first drop of blood should be wiped away.
   d. The tourniquet needs to be tighter than in venipuncture.

78. Which of the following can lead to an increase in the level of enzymes present in the circulation?

   a. Heart damage
   b. Mild exercise

c. Normal diet

d. Rapid change in posture

79. Which of the following is a biologic condition that may affect the results of blood testing?

   a. Diet
   b. Posture
   c. Pregnancy
   d. Trauma

80. Which of the following are part of being a professional?

   a. Dressing appropriately
   b. Being patient
   c. Being well groomed
   d. All of the above

81. The ability to see ourselves as others see us is known as:

   a. Intrapersonal communication
   b. One-way communication
   c. Interpersonal communication
   d. None of the above

82. Which of the following is a barrier to effective communication?

   a. Being a good listener
   b. Both parties paying attention
   c. Mutual understanding
   d. Reference gap

83. Which of the following is true?

   a. A phlebotomist must use both verbal and nonverbal communication.
   b. It is acceptable to show displeasure with a patient when the family is present.
   c. Looking at your watch is an acceptable way to communicate to a patient that you have more work to do.
   d. You should tell a patient if you are a student and just learning.

84. Which of the following IS NOT capital equipment?

   a. Blood pressure cuffs
   b. Centrifuges
   c. Syringes
   d. Timers

85. A(n) _____ is an accounting of expendable supplies.

    a. Capital expenditure program
    b. Inventory
    c. Quality assurance program
    d. Quality control program

86. A prolonged bleeding time is indicative of:

    a. Low platelet count
    b. Low red blood cell count
    c. Low white blood cell count
    d. None of the above

87. Osteomyelitis occurs when:

    a. An infant's heel bone is damaged with a lancet
    b. A patient passes out
    c. A vein collapses
    d. There is swelling from blood leakage around venipuncture site

88. When collecting blood with a syringe, it is best to add the blood to:

    a. The EDTA tube first
    b. The plain red (no anticoagulant) tube first
    c. The sodium citrate tube first
    d. Whichever tube you happen to pick up first

89. Hypoglycemia is a condition consisting of:

    a. High blood glucose level
    b. High cholesterol level
    c. Low blood glucose level
    d. Low cholesterol level

90. Which procedure is generally done by a nurse or respiratory therapist?

    a. Arterial puncture
    b. Glucose tolerance test
    c. Heel stick on an infant
    d. Ivy bleeding time

91. Prepping the puncture site for this procedure is similar to that used for blood donor collection:

    a. Blood culture collections
    b. Duke bleeding time

c. Earlobe microcapillary puncture
d. Routine phlebotomy

92. Which test will require the phlebotomist to perform routine venipuncture but use a special collection tube provided by the manufacturer?

a. Blood donor phlebotomy
b. Clotting time
c. Fibrin degradation products
d. Therapeutic phlebotomy

93. Which of the factors generally DOES NOT contribute to syncope?

a. Cardiac arrhythmia
b. Fatigue
c. Hyperglycemia
d. Sudden decrease in blood volume

94. Which of the following is probably the most common complication from phlebotomy?

a. Convulsions
b. Fainting
c. Hematoma
d. Hyperventilation

95. A collapsed vein may result in:

a. Convulsions
b. Hematoma
c. Hypovolemia
d. Short draw

96. Which of the following is a technical error in phlebotomy?

a. Convulsions
b. Fainting
c. Hematoma
d. Missing a vein

97. Which of the following occurrences IS NOT a cause for specimen rejection?

a. Clot in a "tiger top" tube
b. Clot in an EDTA tube
c. Hemolysis in a blood bank specimen
d. Short draw in sodium citrate tube

98. Which area of the laboratory often has the strictest specimen collection requirements?

    a. Bacteriology
    b. Blood bank
    c. Chemistry
    d. Hematology

99. This virus accounts for the majority of post-transfusion cases of hepatitis in the United States.

    a. Hepatitis A virus
    b. Hepatitis B virus
    c. Hepatitis C virus
    d. Hepatitis delta virus

100. This recent OSHA regulation requires that all health care personnel at risk for exposure to _____ receive vaccination.

    a. Hepatitis A virus
    b. Hepatitis B virus
    c. Hepatitis C virus
    d. Hepatitis delta virus

Answers

1.	C	16.	B	31.	D	46.	D	61.	B
2.	B	17.	D	32.	C	47.	B	62.	B
3.	A	18.	B	33.	B	48.	B	63.	A
4.	C	19.	D	34.	C	49.	C	64.	A
5.	A	20.	B	35.	B	50.	A	65.	B
6.	B	21.	D	36.	A	51.	B	66.	C
7.	A	22.	D	37.	B	52.	C	67.	A
8.	A	23.	A	38.	B	53.	C	68.	D
9.	C	24.	A	39.	D	54.	D	69.	A
10.	C	25.	C	40.	C	55.	C	70.	A
11.	D	26.	B	41.	B	56.	D	71.	D
12.	D	27.	B	42.	A	57.	B	72.	A
13.	A	28.	A	43.	C	58.	A	73.	B
14.	B	29.	A	44.	A	59.	B	74.	C
15.	D	30.	B	45.	B	60.	D	75.	C

76.	D	81.	A	86.	A	91.	A	96.	D
77.	C	82.	D	87.	A	92.	C	97.	A
78.	A	83.	A	88.	C	93.	C	98.	B
79.	C	84.	C	89.	C	94.	C	99.	C
80.	D	85.	B	90.	A	95.	D	100.	B

Index

Note: Page numbers in *italics* indicate figures; those followed by t indicate tables.

233